A Guide to Gastrointestinal Motility Disorders

Albert J. Bredenoord • André Smout
Jan Tack

A Guide to Gastrointestinal Motility Disorders

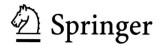 Springer

Albert J. Bredenoord
Gastroenterology and Hepatology
Academic Medical Centre
Amsterdam, The Netherlands

Jan Tack
Gastroenterology and Hepatology
UZ Leuven
Leuven, Belgium

André Smout
Gastroenterology and Hepatology
Academic Medical Centre
Amsterdam, The Netherlands

The work was first published in 2010 by Bohn Stafleu van Loghum with the following title: "Functiestoornissen van het maag-darmkanaal" by Arjan Bredenoord, Jan Tack, André Smout - ISBN print: 978-90-313-7839-5

ISBN 978-3-319-26936-8   ISBN 978-3-319-26938-2   (eBook)
DOI 10.1007/978-3-319-26938-2

Library of Congress Control Number: 2016930027

Springer Cham Heidelberg New York Dordrecht London

Printed on acid-free paper

Springer International Publishing AG Switzerland is part of Springer Science+Business Media
(www.springer.com)

Contents

Functional Anatomy and Physiology

1.1 Introduction

The gastrointestinal tract can be regarded as a hollow tube divided into several compartments. Each compartment has its own structure, related to its function. We distinguish the esophagus, stomach, small bowel, and large bowel or colon. Glands produce juices that play an important role in digestion, the salivary glands produce saliva, the stomach secretes hydrochloric acid and pepsin, the liver produces bile, and the pancreas produces amylase, lipase, and tryptase. The various compartments differ in diameter and are delimited by sphincters that open and close at the correct moments (Fig. 1.1).

This allows the partly digested food or feces to be expelled in the right direction. The wall of the compartments of the gastrointestinal tract is different for each compartment; however, the basic structure is similar.

1.2 The Basic Structure

The wall consists of several layers (Fig. 1.2). From the inner to the outer layers, there is the mucosa, submucosa, muscularis propria, and serosa (Fig. 1.3).

1.2.1 The Mucosa

The mucosa forms the barrier between the luminal content and the internal environment. The mucosa consists of the epithelium, a thin muscular layer of smooth muscle (muscularis mucosae), and in between the connective tissue of the lamina propria.

1.2.2 The Submucosa

The submucosa mainly consists of fibrous tissue. In this layer a network of nerve cells is found, the submucosal plexus.

1.2.3 The Muscularis Propria

The muscularis propria surrounds the submucosa. The muscularis propria consists of an inner longitudinal muscular layer and an outer circular muscular layer. In between the two muscular layers, a nervous network exists called the myenteric plexus that plays an important role in regulation and coordination of the contractions of these muscular layers.

© Springer International Publishing Switzerland 2016
A.J. Bredenoord et al., *A Guide to Gastrointestinal Motility Disorders*,
DOI 10.1007/978-3-319-26938-2_1

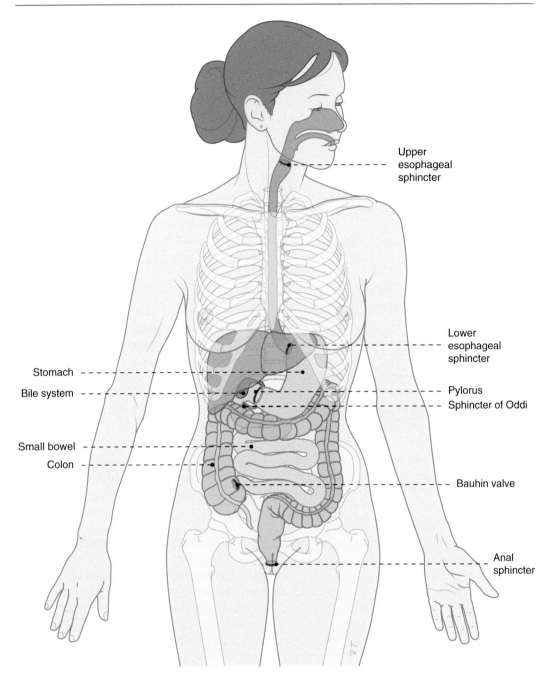

Fig. 1.1 Schematic display of the different compartments and sphincters of the gastrointestinal tract. Each compartment is divided from the previous and following compartment by sphincters (Published with kind permission of © Rogier Trompert Medical Art 2015)

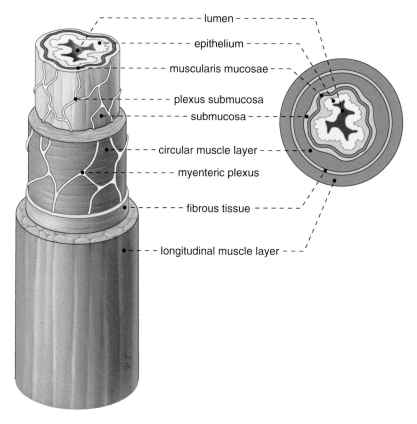

lumen
epithelium
muscularis mucosae
plexus submucosa
submucosa
circular muscle layer
myenteric plexus
fibrous tissue
longitudinal muscle layer

Fig. 1.2 Schematic figure of the different layers of the gastrointestinal tract (Published with kind permission of © Rogier Trompert Medical Art 2015)

1.2.4   The Serosa

The serosa is the outer layer of the gastrointestinal tract and consists of fibrous tissue. In the serosa blood vessels, lymph vessels, and nerve fibers are present. In contrast to the other parts of the digestive canal, the esophagus does not have a serosa.

1.3   The Esophagus

The esophagus is a muscular tube that connects the pharynx with the stomach. Its function is to transport food and saliva from the mouth to the stomach and to prevent reflux of gastric contents. The structure and function of the esophagus are closely connected.

The mucosa of the esophagus consists of multiple layers of squamous epithelium. The transition from esophageal to gastric mucosa is normally in the distal esophagus. It is sometimes called the z-line because of its z-shaped appearance that one can find during endoscopy. The esophagus does not play a role in absorption of food and liquids and its lining is relatively smooth.

The upper and lower esophageal sphincters seal off the esophagus from the pharynx and stomach. The upper esophageal sphincter consists of striated muscle, and the lower esophageal sphincter consists of smooth muscle. In the tubular esophagus, between the two sphincters, one can find these two kinds of muscle fibers. The proximal third consists of striated muscle and the distal two-thirds consist of smooth muscle.

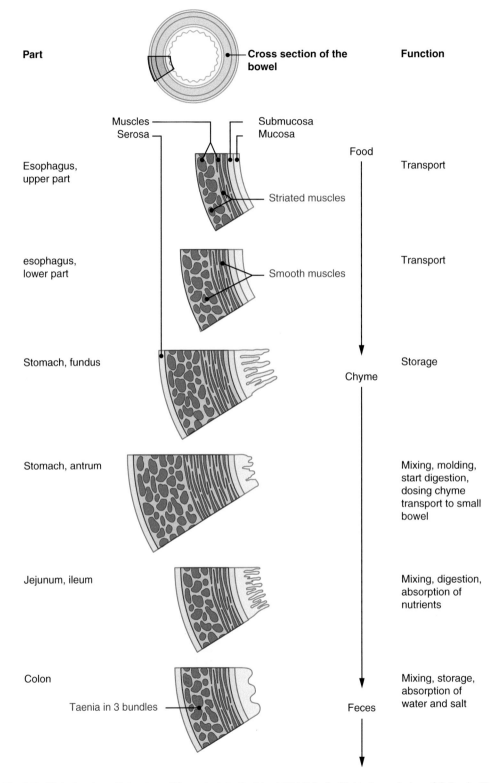

Fig. 1.3 Variations in wall structure of the gastrointestinal tract (Published with kind permission of © Rogier Trompert Medical Art 2015)

1.4   The Stomach

The stomach is a bag-shaped organ bordered by the lower esophageal sphincter and the pylorus. The pylorus connects the stomach with the small bowel. A distinction in function can be made between the fundus and antrum and in between the body of the stomach. The fundus serves as a temporary storage for food until it can be grinded in the antrum.

The gastric mucosa has many folds, in order to create a large surface. The gastric mucosa consists of a singular layer of cylindrical epithelial cells. In the epithelium mucus is produced that protects the cells against the acidic gastric contents. In the body of the stomach, there are gland tubes with parietal cells and gastric chief cells. Parietal cells produce acid and intrinsic factor, and chief cells produce pepsinogen, the precursor of the protein-digesting enzyme pepsin.

The gastric muscle layer is rather thick, in particular in the antrum. Proximally an extra muscle layer is present below the circular muscle layers. This extra muscle layer consists of diagonal muscle fibers and allows creation of a tonical pressure in the stomach.

1.5   The Small Bowel

The small bowel is the longest part of the gastrointestinal tract and measures about 5 m in total. The duodenum is about 25 cm long and is followed by 2 m of jejunum and 3 m of ileum. The small bowel starts at the pylorus and ends at the ileocecal valve (valve of Bauhin), where the small bowel empties in the colon.

The small bowel mucosa consists of a single layer of cylindrical epithelium and is even much more folded than in the stomach. The folds and villi increase the surface of the 5 m long small bowel up to the surface of a soccer field, which allows intensive transportation of nutrients through and along epithelial cells. The most important function of the small bowel is the uptake of these nutrients. The muscle layers of the small bowel are much thinner than the muscle layers of the distal stomach. The serosa of the

small bowel is attached to the mesentery. The position of the small bowel is very flexible, and only the duodenum and ileocolonic valve are fixated.

1.6   The Colon

The colon is about one-and-a-half meter long and is also called large bowel because of its diameter. The colon starts at the ileocolonic valve and ends at the anal canal. We differentiate the cecum, ascending colon, transverse colon, descending colon, sigmoid, and rectum. Also in the colon, a single layer of cylindrical epithelium is found. The colonic wall is not folded and is relatively flat, and surface enhancement is realized with crypts. The organization of the muscle layers of the colon is a variation of the overall structure of the gastrointestinal tract. The inner circular muscle layer contracts at intervals, and these are called haustrations and give the colon its typical shape. The outer longitudinal muscle layer is organized into three bundles called taeniae. Between the taeniae there are virtually no longitudinal fibers present. The function of the colon is absorption of electrolytes and water which results in the feces becoming more solid.

1.7   The Anorectum

The rectum is the continuation of the colon but differs from it considerably in structure and function. The longitudinal muscle layers of the rectum are not organized in bundles but are continuous, and the rectum is covered by the peritoneum. The function of the rectum is storage of feces until it is defecated. The rectum ends at the anal canal. The anal canal is 2–4 cm long and is lined proximally by a single layer of cylindrical epithelium and distally by anoderm. The transition from cylindrical epithelium to anoderm is zipper or teeth shaped and is therefore sometimes called dentate line or linea dentata. The most important function of the anus is to maintain continence, and this is brought about by the smooth muscles of the internal anal sphincter and the striated muscles of the external anal sphincter. In addition to this, the muscles of the pelvic floor play an important role in continence as well.

1.8   The Gallbladder and Bile Ducts

The production of bile from the liver flows through the bile ducts to the intestine (Fig. 1.4).

The left and right hepatic ducts merge at the level of the liver hilum and together form the common bile duct. The cystic duct branches off from the common bile duct a bit more distally and connects the gallbladder. Distally, the bile duct enters the pancreas and merges with the pancreatic duct into the papilla of Vater. The most distal part of the bile duct is surrounded by smooth muscle that serves as a sphincter, and this is called the sphincter of Oddi. This sphincter regulates the flow of bile into the duodenum and prevents migration of bacteria into the bile ducts. When there are no nutrients within the gut, the bile flows into the gallbladder and is stored temporarily. The wall of the gallbladder consists of muscle fibers which make that the gallbladder can contract and squeeze its contents through the bile ducts toward the duodenum. The epithelium of the gallbladder and bile ducts consists of a single layer of cylindrical epithelium. Active reabsorption of water from the bile takes place in the gallbladder, which leads to concentration of the bile. The function of bile is facilitation of digestion and absorption of food in the intestines.

1.9   Nerves

The gastrointestinal system has its own nervous system that can function independently of the central nervous system. This nervous system is called the enteric nervous system and is found in the wall of all organs of the gastrointestinal tract. The enteric nervous system is influenced by sympathetic and parasympathetic fibers of the autonomous nervous system (Fig. 1.5).

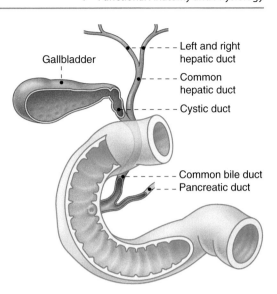

Fig. 1.4 Overview of bile ducts and gallbladder (Published with kind permission of © Rogier Trompert Medical Art 2015)

The activity of the gastrointestinal tract is not directly controlled by the mind. Only at the beginning and the end we can influence activity of the muscles of the gastrointestinal tract by swallowing and defecation. The gastrointestinal tract is thus intrinsically controlled by the enteric nervous system and extrinsically by the autonomous nervous system and a limited number of other nerves. Hormones also play an important role in the regulation of digestion.

1.9.1   The Enteric Nervous System

The enteric nervous system consists of networks of nervous cells in the wall of the gastrointestinal tract. The enteric nervous system functions independently of the central nervous system and controls movements, secretion, and microcirculation of the gastrointestinal tract. The cell bodies of the nervous cells are located in the myenteric plexus and submucosal plexus. The myenteric plexus is found between the circular and longitudinal muscle layers of the bowels and provides control of the motor neurons of these muscle layers. The submucosal plexus is found in the submucosa. It is further divided in an inner plexus,

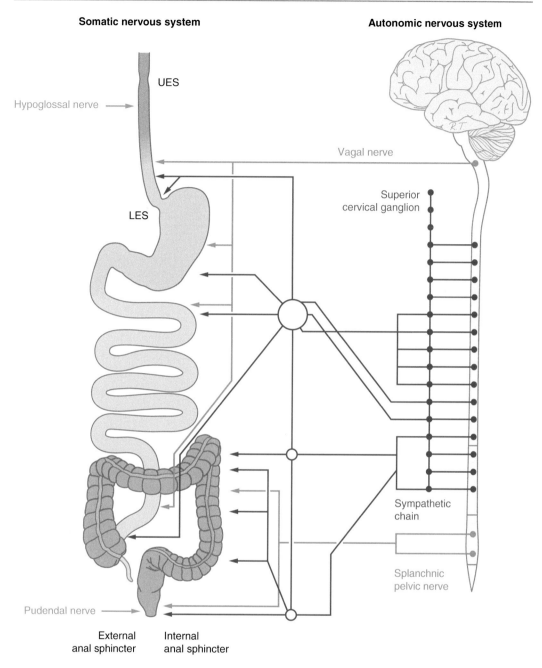

Fig. 1.5 Schematic overview of the nerves of the gastrointestinal tract (Published with kind permission of © Rogier Trompert Medical Art 2015)

close to the mucosa, which controls secretion and an outer plexus, closer to the muscle layers, which is involved in control of motility.

The enteric nervous system is found in each part of the gastrointestinal tract, from the esophagus to anus. The nerves of the pancreas, gallblad-

der, and bile ducts are also under control of the enteric nervous system.

Neurotransmission in the enteric nervous system is complex, and there are more than 30 different neurotransmitters known to be involved in the regulation of the gastrointestinal tract. The most important neurotransmitters are acetylcho-line, nitric oxide (NO), serotonin, noradrenalin, somatostatin, substance P, and cholecystokinin (CCK). The number of nerve cells in the enteric nervous system is more than ten million, which is even more than nerve cells in the spinal cord! This is the reason why the enteric nervous system is sometimes referred to as "the little brain."

The enteric nervous system communicates with the central nervous system using the autonomous nervous system.

1.9.2 The Role of the Autonomous Nervous System

The autonomous nervous system consists of the sympathetic and parasympathetic innervation. Overall, the parasympathetic influence stimulates the motility and secretion of the gastrointestinal tract, while the sympathetic system inhibits its activity.

1.9.2.1 The Parasympathetic Nerves

The parasympathetic nerve fibers run directly from the spinal cord to the myenteric and submucosal plexus, where they form synapses with the enteric nervous system. The most important neurotransmitter of the parasympathetic system is acetylcholine. The most important parasympathetic nerve is the vagus nerve or the tenth cranial nerve. The cell bodies of this nerve are within the brain stem. The nerve fibers run along the esophagus and reach the abdomen through the same opening in the diaphragm through which the esophagus goes. Most fibers of the vagus nerve are afferent (sensory) nerves that pass information on from the gastrointestinal tract to the central nervous system. These fibers have endings at the proximal part of the gastrointestinal tract. The parasympathetic innervation of the distal colon and rectum goes through fibers of the pelvic splanchnic nerves that exit the spinal cord at sacral level.

1.9.2.2 The Sympathetic Nerves

The cell bodies of the sympathetic nerves are at the thoracolumbar level of the spinal cord. They run through paravertebral ganglia to the preverte-bral ganglia, which are the celiac ganglion, superior mesenteric ganglion, and inferior mesenteric ganglion. From these ganglia the fibers follow the mesenteric arteries and reach the bowels. The most important neurotransmitter of this system is noradrenalin.

1.9.3 The Role of Nerves under Voluntary Control

The movements of the mouth, throat, and upper esophageal sphincter are controlled voluntarily. The hypoglossal nerve (twelfth cranial nerve) innervates the striated muscles of hypopharynx and upper esophageal sphincter and coordinates swallowing. The external anal sphincter also consists of striated muscle and is also controlled voluntarily via the pudendal nerve. This allows timing of defecation.

1.9.4 The Role of Hormones

In addition to the nervous system, also hormones play an important role in the regulation of digestion. Some hormones have an inhibitory influence on the activity of the digestive system, while others stimulate its activity. We distinguish endocrine and paracrine effects of hormones. Endocrine hormones are released in the circulation and subsequently reach their target. An example is glucagon. Paracrine secretion refers to a local effect after local secretion, such as occurring with histamine. Some compounds have a role as a hormone *and* as a neurotransmitter.

1.9.5 Separation into Compartments

As mentioned previously, the gastrointestinal tract is separated into compartments, each with a specific structure that is related to its function. These compartments are separated by sphincters whose main function is to prevent retrograde flow of contents from the one compartment to the previous compartment. The lower esophageal sphincter protects reflux of gastric contents into the esophagus, and the ileocecal valve prevents retrograde flow of colonic bacteria into the small bowel. The wall of each compartment resists the contents of that compartment, but contents of other compartments may damage it. Furthermore, the separation into compartments allows homeostasis of the compartments. The protein-digesting enzyme pepsin is only active in the acidic environment of the stomach, while the enzyme trypsin that splices proteins in the duodenum is only active in an alkaline environment. The pylorus makes it possible that the acidity of the stomach (pH = 2) is much lower than the acidity of the duodenum (pH = 7–8) which allows the activity of these enzymes in each of their compartments.

1.10   Contractility and Motility of the Gastrointestinal Tract

The movements of the gastrointestinal tract are mainly caused by smooth muscles. Only the upper esophageal sphincter, the proximal esophagus, and the external anal sphincter consist of striated muscle. Smooth muscle fibers are different from striated muscle because the first can contract in a prolonged (tonic) fashion and are not under voluntary control. We distinguish phasic and tonic contractions of smooth muscles. The phasic contractions are short lasting and often rhythmic, and the tonic contractions are prolonged. In the proximal stomach, gallbladder, and sphincters, there are mainly tonic contractions; in the esophagus, distal stomach, and small bowel, mainly phasic contractions occur. In the colon both phasic and tonic contractions have an important role.

1.10.1   The Rhythm of the Stomach and Intestines

Smooth muscle cells are negatively electrically charged, which means there is a potential difference across their cell membrane. This potential difference is not constant but varies cyclically. The potential difference increases until a depolarization takes place. The cell remains depolarized

for a few seconds, after which the cycle repeats itself. This cycle is independent of whether or not the smooth muscle cell contracts. This activity is referred to as basic electrical rhythm, as slow waves, or as electrical control activity. The frequency of this rhythm is 3/min in the stomach, 12/min in duodenum, and 9/min in the terminal ileum. The basal rhythmic activity starts in the interstitial cells of Cajal, specialized nerve cells that serve as a pacemaker. These cells are grouped in pacemaker regions. In the stomach this region is located proximally at the larger curvature, and in the duodenum several pacemaker regions are scattered in the intestinal wall. The cells of Cajal pass the rhythm on to the smooth muscle cells that further pass it on distally.

In addition to the basal electrical rhythm, there is a second type of electrical activity, which is called spike activity or action potential. These action potentials are initiated by motor neurons of the enteric nervous system. Once acetylcholine is released by these motor neurons, muscarinic receptors on the smooth muscle cells are activated, and calcium ions flow into the cell. If this occurs during the depolarization phase, it leads to a contraction of the muscle cell. The motor neurons are influenced by hormones, the autonomous nervous system, and other neurons of the enteric nervous system. Because action potentials can only be generated in the depolarized state, the basal rhythmic activity determines when a muscle cell can contract. Because the phase of the basal rhythmic activity is propagated in distal direction, the phasic contraction will do likewise.

1.10.2   From Contraction to Peristalsis

When phasic contractions of the smooth muscle layers are propagated in distal direction, it is called peristalsis. The peristaltic reflex, triggered by stretch of the bowel wall, ensures transport of bowel contents (bolus) (Fig. 1.6).

Stretch activates mechanoreceptors in the bowel wall that pass a signal to the enteric nervous system. The segment distal of the segment in which stretch was perceived will relax in order to anticipate on the bolus' arrival. The segment proximal to the segment in which the stretch was perceived will contract in order to propel the bolus. The result is that the bolus that causes the

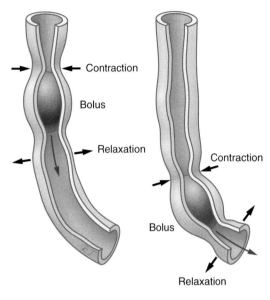

stretch is moved in distal direction. The enteric nervous system coordinates this peristaltic movement.

1.10.3 Tonic Contractions

A tonic contraction is a prolonged contraction of a muscle that lasts for minutes up to hours. Tonic contractions are found everywhere in the gastro-intestinal tract and are responsible for a certain pressure in the lumen. Tonic contractions and relaxations are mainly important in organs that serve as a temporal storage, such as the proximal stomach, the gallbladder, and the rectum.

1.10.4 Digestion

Once food is seen or smelled, preparations for digestion are started. The secretion of saliva is stimulated and the stomach begins to contract and secrete its juices. Once the eating starts, the proximal stomach relaxes in order to accommodate the food without increasing intragastric pressure. This phenomenon is called adaptive relaxation (Fig. 1.7).

Fig. 1.6 Schematic representation of a peristaltic wave. Proximal to the bolus, a contraction occurs and distal to the bolus relaxation occurs. The result is movement of the bolus in distal direction (Published with kind permission of © Rogier Trompert Medical Art 2015)

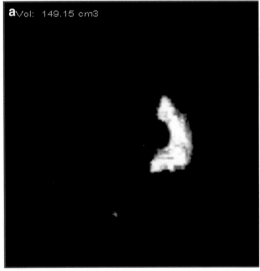
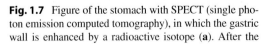
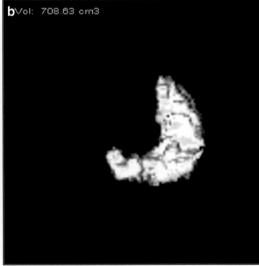

Fig. 1.7 Figure of the stomach with SPECT (single photon emission computed tomography), in which the gastric wall is enhanced by a radioactive isotope (**a**). After the meal (**b**) there is a large increase in gastric volume as a result of adaptive relaxation

Stretch of the stomach by the swallowed food and the presence of nutrients will further stimulate gastric acid production. Soon after the first food has entered the stomach, phasic contractions start with a frequency of 3/min. The contractions in the distal stomach grind the food and finally transport it to the duodenum. Bile and pancreatic juices flow into the duodenum and mix with the food bolus and facilitate digestion and solubility of the nutrients. The small bowel will transport the bolus in smaller volumes in distal direction. The speed at which the stomach empties is dependent on the volume and type of food. Complete emptying of the stomach usually requires 3 h. The passage through the small bowel, from the pylorus to colon, takes around 90 min. The presence in the colon is extremely variable.

1.10.5 The Intestines Between Meals

When all digestible food has emptied from the stomach, the fed state pattern of motility and secretion stops and switches to the interdigestive pattern (Fig. 1.8).

The interdigestive starts with a phase I, characterized by a complete inactivity of the stomach. This phase lasts for approximately 40 min. After these peristaltic waves are gradually appearing, this is phase II. This phase also lasts for about 40 min. During phase II the proportion of depolarizations associated with contractions is increasing. In phase III the contractions have reached a maximal amplitude and frequency, in the stomach this is three per minute. The pressure of the lower esophageal sphincter is also maximal. In the small bowel, the frequency of contractions has reached 12/min. After 10 min of phase III activity, the contractions decrease until the stomach is in the complete quiescence of phase I again, and the cycle repeats itself. This 90 min cycle of activity between meals is called the migrating motor complex (MMC). The aim of the MMC is to get rid of indigestible remains of foods and to prevent stasis of bacteria. During phase III there is also maximal secretion of gastric juice, bile, and pancreatic juices. The forceful peristaltic contractions during phase III together with the secreted juices flush and clean the stomach and intestines, and therefore, the MMC is sometimes called *housekeeping* activity of the bowel.

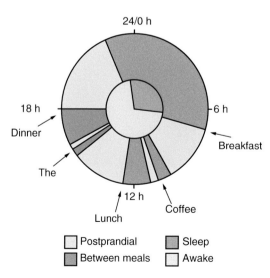

Fig. 1.8 Example of the phases of the gastrointestinal tract. Food intake determines whether the gastrointestinal tract is in the fed state or interdigestive state (Published with kind permission of © Rogier Trompert Medical Art 2015)

1.11   Functional Disorders of the Gastrointestinal Tract

Functional disorders of the gastrointestinal tract are disorders characterized by symptoms suggestive of a cause within the gastrointestinal tract, while there are no visible, histopathological, or otherwise objectifiable abnormalities demonstrable. However, in case of the most prevalent functional bowel disorders such as functional dyspepsia and irritable bowel syndrome, more and more data from scientific research suggests that objectifiable abnormalities are present that could explain the symptoms of these patients. Abnormalities in motility, sensation, permeability, inflammation, and secretion are all found. Stress seems to play an important role in triggering these disorders (Fig. 1.9).

These abnormalities cannot be used yet for diagnostic purposes of functional bowel disorders.

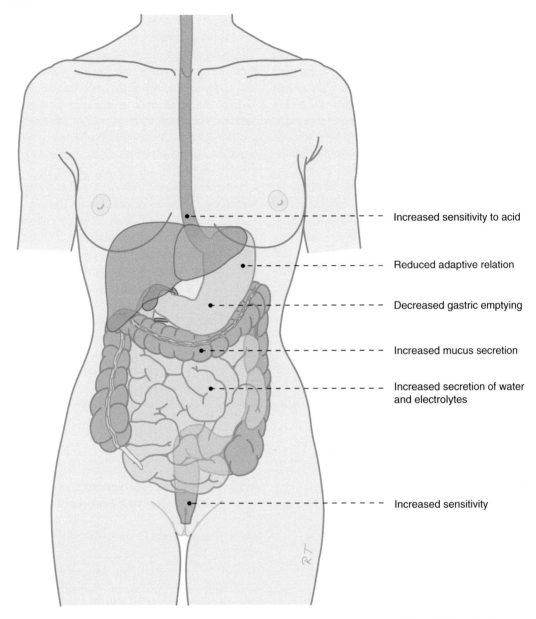

Increased sensitivity to acid

Reduced adaptive relation

Decreased gastric emptying

Increased mucus secretion

Increased secretion of water and electrolytes

Increased sensitivity

Fig. 1.9 The influence of stress on the gastrointestinal tract (Published with kind permission of © Rogier Trompert Medical Art 2015)

The reason is that there is a considerable overlap with healthy subjects without symptoms.

1.11.1 Classification of Functional Disorders: The Road to Rome

Classically, a diagnosis is made when a well-defined measurable or visible abnormality is found that does not occur in healthy subjects. In functional disorders the diagnosis is based on the presence of a specific combination of symptoms, in the absence of an alternative explanation for the symptoms. For a long time, functional disorders were mainly defined by what they were not, and as a consequence of the lack of a clear definition, there were large differences in what people meant with a certain condition. This complicated discussions among doctors and made interpretation of scientific study results difficult. One of the first attempts to define a functional disorder is the Manning criteria for the diagnosis of the irritable bowel syndrome. In 1988 a group of international experts aiming to define all functional disorders of the gastrointestinal tract met in Rome. This resulted in the publication of the Rome criteria in 1994, later followed by the Rome II criteria in 1999, the Rome III criteria in 2006, and the most recent Rome IV criteria in 2015. In the Rome criteria, all functional disorders of the gastrointestinal tract are organized and defined based on the presence of frequently occurring combinations of symptoms. The Rome criteria have led to uniform definitions of these disorders and have made exchange and interpretation of information much easier.

2.1 Introduction

The diagnosis of disorders of gastrointestinal motility and functional disorders of the gastrointestinal tract can be facilitated by various investigational techniques. The most important of these will be discussed in this chapter.

2.2 Manometry

Measurement of the pressure (manometry) in the lumen of the gastrointestinal canal is an important aid in the study of the motor patterns of the canal. The most commonly used types of manometry allow the detection and quantification of the phasic contractions of the wall of the digestive tube. In addition, specialized forms of manometry can be utilized to record the tonic tone in sphincters and relaxations of sphincters.

An important principle is that a contraction of the gut wall is associated with a measurable increase in intraluminal pressure only if the contraction leads to a closed compartment in which a pressure rise can occur. Contractions that do not occlude the lumen do not lead to a measurable pressure increase. Thus, manometry can fail to lead to meaningful results when it is applied to organs that are wide, such as the proximal part of the stomach or the colon, or in a part of the digestive tract that has become distended during the course of a disease process (such as intestinal pseudo-obstruction). In fact, the majority of phasic contractions of the digestive tract will not lead to compartmentalization and thus not to a measurable pressure rise.

2.2.1 Perfused versus Solid-State Manometry

Basically, there are two different ways of measuring pressures in the lumen of the gastrointestinal canal (Fig. 2.1). With the first of these, a multi-lumen catheter is used, the channels of which are each perfused with water (water-perfused manometry). The water that runs through the individual water channels exits the catheter through side holes. Thus, perfused manometric systems measure pressure in one direction of the circumference. In water perfusion manometry, the pressure in the lumen of the gut is transferred, via the water in the individual channels, to pressure transducers outside the human body. The conversion of the pressure in each of the water-perfused channels to electrical signal takes place outside the body. For the perfusion of the water channels in the catheter, specialized systems are used that ensure a low and constant perfusion speed (between 0.08 and 0.3 ml/min). These so-called minimally compliant perfusion systems make it possible that the perfusion speed is not affected by pressure changes. This allows reliable pressure recording.

© Springer International Publishing Switzerland 2016
A.J. Bredenoord et al., *A Guide to Gastrointestinal Motility Disorders*,
DOI 10.1007/978-3-319-26938-2_2

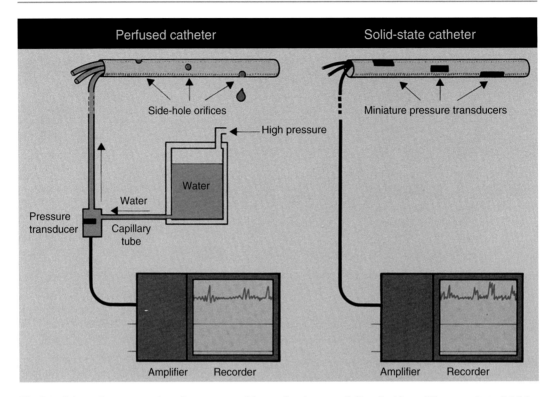

Fig. 2.1 Schematic representation of manometry with a perfused system (*left*) and with a solid-state catheter (*right*)

The recording of pressures exerted at side holes in a perfused manometric catheter assembly is useful for the study of peristaltic sequences in tubular parts of the digestive tract (e.g., esophageal peristalsis) but has clear limitations when the motor functions of a sphincter are to be studied. Movements, such as caused by respiration or shortening, make the pressure sensor slip in and out of the sphincter, leading to a pressure signal that is difficult to interpret. In order to solve this problem, the Australian gastroenterologist John Dent developed the so-called sleeve sensor. The sleeve sensor consists of a 5–6-cm-long membrane mounted on the manometric catheter. Water runs underneath the sleeve. The highest pressure exerted at any point on the sleeve is recorded. The Dent sleeve is particularly useful for pressure recording from the lower esophageal sphincter (LES). With the advent of high-resolution manometry, the sleeve sensor has become less indispensable, since high-resolution manometry also makes it possible to record sphincter pressures in a reliable way. This will be discussed below (Fig. 2.2).

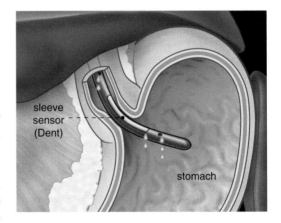

Fig. 2.2 Sleeve catheter, positioned in the lower esophageal sphincter (Published with kind permission of © Rogier Trompert Medical Art 2015)

Basal pressure in a sphincter (tone) can also be measured by pulling the manometric catheter through the sphincter while continuously recording the pressure ("pull-through technique").

The second method for manometry in the gastrointestinal canal uses miniature pressure sensors mounted in or on a catheter. No water perfusion is used with this so-called "solid-state" method. Each of the pressure sensors in the catheter converts the pressure to which it is exposed to an electrical signal. Because water perfusion is not needed, the solid-state technique can be used much more easily for pressure recording in ambulatory subjects. This offers advantages when prolonged manometry is to be carried out (e.g., to detect esophageal spasm in patients with noncardiac chest pain or to study small bowel dysmotility in patients with (suspected) intestinal pseudo-obstruction).

The advantages of water-perfused manometry are that the catheters are relatively cheap and very durable. A disadvantage is that it can be time-consuming to make the manometric system ready for use, because the water flow through all perfused channels has to be constant and there may be no air bubbles in the system.

Disadvantages of the solid-state manometry are the high price of the catheters and their vulnerability. Its enormous advantage is the ease of performance of the manometric investigation.

2.2.2   High-Resolution Manometry

The development of *high-resolution* manometry has revolutionized manometric practice, in particular that of esophageal manometry. In high-resolution manometry, pressures are measured at closely spaced sites along the manometric catheter. The distance between the sensors typically is 1 cm but can even be smaller. High-resolution manometry can be carried out with a perfused multichannel catheter (and an array of perfused external pressure transducers) or with a solid-state catheter. The latter has gained enormous popularity, in particular in the form of 36-channel esophageal manometry. A 96-channel manometric technique using fiber-optic technology has also been developed but is as yet not commercially available. When a 36-channel catheter with sensors at 1-cm intervals is used, the catheter simultaneously "sees" all relevant structures, namely, the UES, the esophageal body, and the LES. This makes correct positioning of the cath-

eter easy, allowing the manometric procedure to be performed by a less experienced person.

When 36 or more pressure signals are recorded, it becomes difficult to overview all signals. Conventional line plots (with time on the horizontal axis and amplitude on the vertical) fall short in providing a clear overview (Fig. 2.3). Therefore, other ways of representing the data were sought for. Universally, color plots are utilized in which amplitudes are expressed as color (Fig. 2.4). This type of representation is also referred to as "pressure topography" or as "Clouse plots," named after the investigator who pioneered this, the late Ray Clouse.

Obviously, high-resolution manometry can be applied to all parts of the digestive canal. In clinical practice, application in the esophagus and its sphincters has gained most popularity, but high-resolution anorectal manometry has also become standard in many centers (Fig. 2.5).

2.3   pH Recording

Recording of intraluminal pH is mostly done in the esophageal body and less frequently in the stomach. In most parts of the world, esophageal pH monitoring is done most often with a miniature pH electrode mounted on a flexible catheter. Such a catheter is introduced via the nose and positioned at a predefined position. For esophageal pH monitoring, the electrode is usually placed at 5 cm above the upper border of the LES. The catheter is taped to the nose and attached to a portable digital data recorder (Fig. 2.6). The recorder usually is worn at a belt or on a shoulder strap.

In most cases, the measurement is carried out as an outpatient procedure and lasts 24 h or more. It is essential that the patient records all symptom episodes (e.g., heartburn) that occur during the measurement, by pressing an event marker button on the portable data recorder and also by filling in a paper symptom diary.

Catheters for pH recording come into three types. Firstly, a glass pH electrode can be used. There is no doubt that glass electrodes yield the best quality, but they are more bulky than the other types and cannot be sterilized. Secondly, catheters with an antimony pH electrode are available. The technical specifications of antimony electrodes are clearly inferior to those of pH electrodes. An antimony electrode is sensitive not only to the pH of the refluxate but also to other constituents, such as food components. However, antimony electrodes can be produced at low cost, making disposable pH catheters economically viable. Lastly, pH can be measured with an ISFET (ion-sensitive field effective transistor) electrode. The performance of ISFET pH electrodes is almost as good as that of glass pH electrodes. ISFET pH electrodes can also be marketed at prices compatible with disposable use.

It is also possible to measure esophageal pH without a transnasal catheter. Catheter-free pH monitoring employs a capsule containing a pH electrode (antimony) and a radio transmitter. The capsule is placed in the esophagus using a specialized introducer and attached to the esophageal mucosa by penetrating it with a metal pin (Fig. 2.7). The signals transmitted by the capsule are received by an external receiver-storage device, which needs to be in close proximity of the body. The system, consisting of capsule, receiver, and signal analysis software, is marketed as Bravo. The most recent versions of the system allow recording for at least 48 h, which has been shown to be advantageous for diagnosis. The advantage of the pH capsule is that transnasal intubation is avoided. However, some patients experience intolerable retrosternal discomfort or pain once the capsule is placed. The costs associated with capsule pH monitoring are higher than those associated with catheter-based pH monitoring.

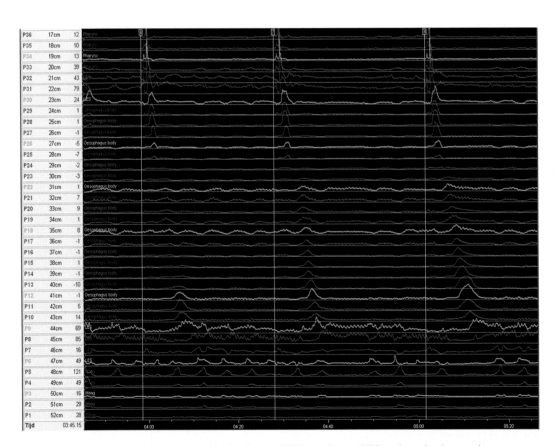

Fig. 2.3 36-channel recording of pressures in the pharynx, UES, esophagus, LES, and proximal stomach

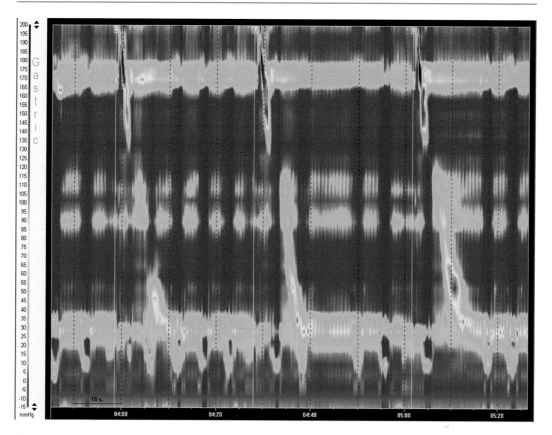

Fig. 2.4   Same 36 pressure signals as in Fig. 2.3 but now represented as color plot

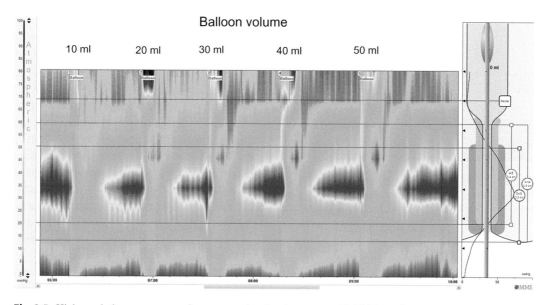

Fig. 2.5   High-resolution manometry of anorectum showing the recto-anal inhibition reflex (relaxation of internal anal sphincter at filling of rectal balloon with 10–50 ml of air)

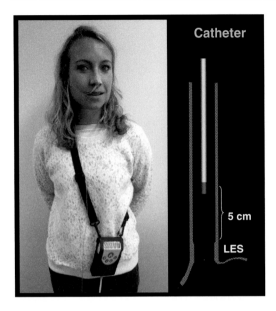

Fig. 2.6 Ambulatory esophageal pH monitoring with a transnasal pH catheter

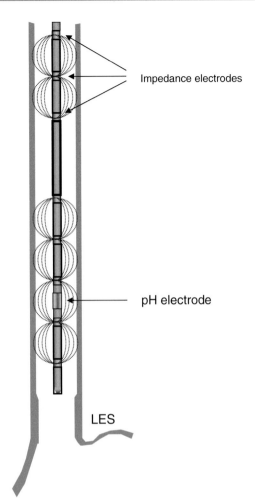

Fig. 2.8 Schematic representation of a catheter with 8 impedance electrodes and one pH electrode, suitable for 24-h reflux monitoring in the esophagus

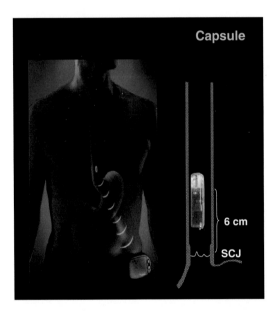

Fig. 2.7 Ambulatory esophageal pH monitoring with a telemetric capsule (*SCJ* squamocolumnar junction, also known as z-line)

2.4   Impedance Monitoring

Electrical impedance is the resistance encountered by an alternating electrical current. The well-known Ohm's law describes resistance to a direct electrical current as the voltage difference across the resistance divided by the current running through it. The resistance is expressed in Ohm (Ω). In the case of an alternating current, the resistance, still expressed in Ω, is composed of not only a resistive but also a capacitive and inductive component, making it dependent of the frequency of the current.

There are several applications of the impedance measurement technique in the human body. One of these is measurement of intraluminal impedance in the digestive canal. For this application a catheter is used on which an array of circular electrodes is mounted (Fig. 2.8). An alternating current that runs from one electrode to the next experiences a resistance (impedance) that depends on what is between the two electrodes. When the current goes through air, it will experience an almost infinitely high impedance. In contrast, when a well-conducting fluid, such as saliva or gastric juice, is between the electrodes, the impedance is low. Using these principles, intraluminal impedance measurement can be used to study the transit of air and fluid through the gastrointestinal canal. The most frequently used application of intraluminal impedance monitoring is in the esophagus.

Esophageal intraluminal impedance monitoring can be used to study the transit of swallowed boluses or to study gastroesophageal reflux. In addition, the technique can be used to study belching and aerophagia, and baseline impedance can be measured as a measure of esophageal integrity. If impedance monitoring is used to assess transit, it is usually combined with pressure recording. For this purpose solid-state high-resolution manometry catheters fitted with impedance electrodes are commercially available.

When impedance monitoring is utilized to study gastroesophageal reflux, this is usually combined with pH monitoring. For this purpose, disposable catheters with an array of impedance ring electrodes and one or two ISFET pH electrodes are commercially available (Fig. 2.8). The usual protocol is to conduct a 24-h study in an outpatient setting. All reflux episodes, whether liquid, gaseous, or mixed, can be detected in the impedance signals, and for each of the reflux episodes, the pH of the refluxate can be determined on the basis of the pH signal.

2.5 SmartPill

The SmartPill capsule is a device that can be swallowed and that measures pH, pressure, and temperature inside the gastrointestinal canal. During the journey of the capsule through the gut, the three signals are continuously relayed by a built-in radio transmitter and received by a portable data recorder outside the body. The

device provides a measure of gastric emptying time because a sharp rise in pH is seen when the capsule exits the stomach (Fig. 2.9). In most cases small bowel transit time can also be measured since the pH drops slightly when the capsule enters the colon. Colonic and whole-gut transit time is marked by the loss of signal when the capsule is excreted. Gastric emptying times and whole-gut transit times measured with the capsule in healthy volunteers correlate well with scintigraphic measurement of the same parameters. The clinical relevance of the pressure measurements provided by the system is not yet apparent.

2.6 Radiographic Examination

Ever since the discovery of the Röntgen rays, radiographic examination of the gastrointestinal tract has not been confined to assessment of the anatomy of the canal but has also been used to study its motor function. Despite the fact that newer imaging techniques (such as MRI) also allow assessment of motor function, Röntgen evaluation is still popular for this purpose. Obviously, the disadvantage of the X-ray evaluation is that prolonged observations are not possible.

When radiography is used to study gastrointestinal motor function and transit, barium sulfate suspension is often used to visualize the tract. For investigations of the esophagus and the stomach, the suspension is swallowed, and for small bowel studies, the contrast medium is injected via a nasoduodenal tube. For examination of the colon and the rectum, the contrast can be injected rectally. For some purposes the so-called double-contrast technique is used in which not only barium suspension but also gas is brought into the canal. The radiopaque suspension sticks to the wall of the organ under study, and the radiolucent air or gas fills the lumen. Using this technique, irregularities of the mucosa can be detected more reliably. For the study of esophageal transit, a solid bolus, such as a piece of bread or a marshmallow, is often used in addition to the liquid contrast medium.

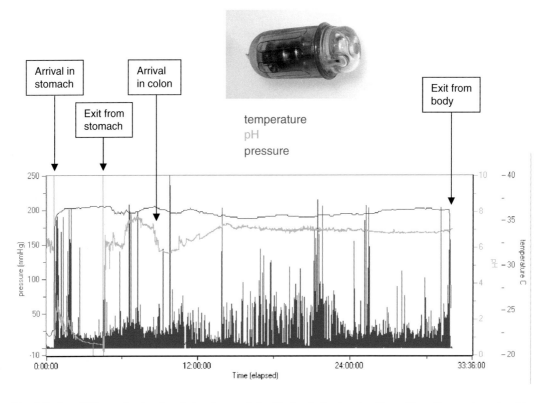

Fig. 2.9 SmartPill capsule (*inset*) and signals recorded with the device in a healthy subject. Temperature signal is shown in *blue*, pH signal in *green*, and pressure signal in *red*

2.6.1 Timed Barium Esophagogram

The timed barium esophagogram technique is a technique to study esophageal emptying in patients with achalasia in a standardized and quantitative way. After ingestion of a standard quantity of barium suspension (usually 150 or 200 ml), anteroposterior radiographic images are obtained at 0, 1, 2, and 5 min. In the picture a ruler is also photographed, allowing for quantitative measurement of height and maximum width of the barium column at each point in time (Fig. 2.10).

2.6.2 Defecography

Defecography is a specialized radiographic technique with which the movements in the anorectal region can be studied, in rest and during defecation. The procedure involves filling of the rectum

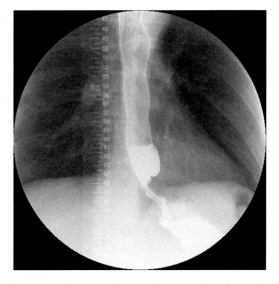

Fig. 2.10 "Timed barium esophagogram." Radiographs of the esophagus are taken at predefined times after ingestion of contrast fluid. A ruler is included in the field

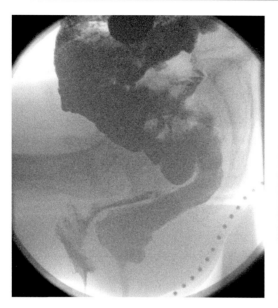

Fig. 2.11 Defecogram. In this lateral picture, one recognizes, from anterior (*left*) to posterior (*right*), the vagina (with some contrast in it), rectum, anus, and coccyx. The array of opaque structures seen posteriorly is a string with metal spheres placed in the perineum

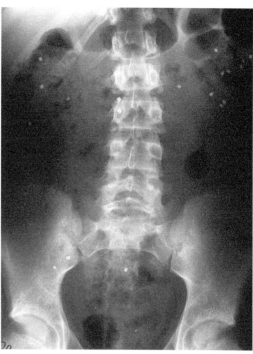

Fig. 2.12 Pellet transit test. Distributed along the colon, the "pellets" are visible as small rings

with a barium sulfate-containing material with a consistency that approaches that of soft feces. The patient is seated on a toilet-like chair. The defecation process is then recorded with X-ray videography using a laterolateral ray path. The images show the movements and the displacements of the rectum, the anal canal, and the pelvic floor that take place during defecation (Fig. 2.11). In the analysis attention is paid to the widening of the anorectal angle that normally takes place during defecation, the descensus of the pelvic floor, the opening of the anal canal, and the expulsion of the contrast medium. In addition, anatomical abnormalities such as a rectocele, enterocele, or intussusception can be visualized. Defecography can also be carried out by magnetic resonance imaging (MRI) technique. Compared to radiography, MRI provides additional anatomical data on pelvic and perineal muscle and other structures. The disadvantages are the recording in a supine position, which is less physiological when studying the act of defecation.

2.6.3 Pellet Transit Test

The pellet transit test is the most often used test to assess the transit time from the mouth to the anus. The patient swallows a number of radiopaque pellets or rings. Subsequently, one or more abdominal X-ray pictures are taken. On these, the number of markers that are still present in the colon is counted. Several variants of this test are in use. The most popular of these is the Hinton test. With this test 20 pellets are ingested on day 0, and an abdominal X-ray is taken on day 5 (approximately 120 h after ingestion of the pellets). On day 5 no more than four pellets should still be visible on the X-ray (Fig. 2.12). If more than four pellets are present on day 5, transit is delayed, and the qualification "slow transit constipation" is applicable. Other variants of the pellet transit test allow estimation of transit time in hours or assessment of regional colonic transit, but the clinical advantage over the simple Hinton test is limited. Because transit through the esophagus, stomach, and small intestine is relatively fast, the pellet transit time largely reflects colonic transit.

2.6.4 Plain Abdominal Radiograph

A plain X-ray of the abdomen, made without administration of a contrast agent, can provide information about the motor functions of the stomach, small intestine, and colon. On a plain abdominal radiograph fluids, air or gas and feces can be distinguished with an adequate level of certainty. On radiographs taken with the patient supine, distended bowel loops and fecal shadowing can be seen. When the radiograph is taken in upright position, air-fluid levels in small and large bowel can be seen when obstruction or pseudo-obstruction is present (Fig. 2.13). Clearly, a plain abdominal radiograph does not provide information on gastrointestinal motility directly, but it reflects the consequences of disordered motility.

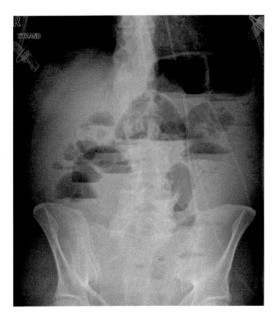

Fig. 2.13 Upright plain abdominal X-ray taken from a patient with intestinal pseudo-obstruction. Air-fluid levels can be seen in the small intestine and colon

2.7 Scintigraphy

Scintigraphic tests, making use of a radioisotope and a gamma camera, can assess transit through the digestive tract. Scintigraphy makes it possible to quantify transit through specific regions in a manner that is minimally distressing the patient. The disadvantage of scintigraphy is that the resolution is not impressive and that a certain amount of ionizing radiation must be administered. The most frequently used scintigraphic technique for the study of gastrointestinal motility is the gastric emptying test. In addition, scintigraphic techniques can be used to assess transit through small bowel and colon and for measurement of bile transport.

2.7.1 Gastric Emptying Test

Scintigraphy is regarded as the gold standard for the measurement of gastric emptying. Many different types of test meals are in use, comprising liquid, solid, and mixed liquid/solid meals. The most frequently used radioactive marker for solid components is technetium-99m (^{99m}Tc). This isotope has a half-life of approximately 6 h. For liquid components the isotope indium-113 (^{113}In) is more suitable, with a half-life of 90 min. When a dual-headed gamma camera is used, the emptying of the solid and liquid fraction of the meal can be measured concurrently. Because the rate of emptying of a meal is dependent on the composition of the meal and its nutritional value, normal values obtained with one specific meal cannot be applied to test results obtained with another meal. Each nuclear medicine department that performs gastric emptying must therefore either establish its own normal values or exactly duplicate the technique developed and validated in another center.

In the analysis of a scintigraphic gastric emptying study, a plot of the activity in the gastric region as a function of time is constructed (Fig. 2.14). In particular with solid meals, there is an initial period of 20 min or so after ingestion of the meal during which no activity leaves the stomach. This phase is known as the "lag phase."

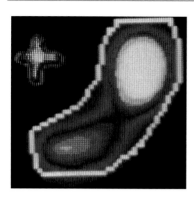
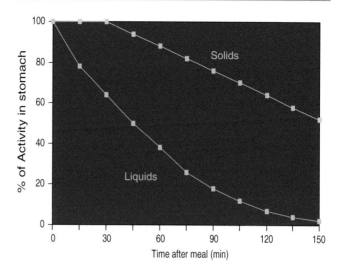

Fig. 2.14 Scintigraphic gastric emptying. *Left panel*: radioactivity in the stomach, as seen by the gamma camera. *Right panel*: time-activity curve of radioactivity in the region of interest

The actual emptying process can be quantified as percentage of ingested activity leaving the stomach per hour or as the retention after 1 and 2 h (expressed as percentage of the ingested dose).

2.7.2   Measurement of Small Intestinal and Colonic Transit Time

After ingestion of a radioactively labeled test meal, the transit of the food through the small intestine can be visualized with a gamma camera, and transit time can be measured. In general, clinicians regard small intestinal transit time of limited interest for patient management. Scintigraphic measurement of colonic transit is not very widely used either. However, scintigraphy does allow one to study not only total colonic but also regional colonic transit.

2.7.3   HIDA Scintigraphy

Scintigraphic techniques can also be used to study bile flow. Most commonly radioactively labeled iminodiacetic acid (IDA) is used for this purpose. The marker is injected intravenously, after which it is excreted within minutes in the bile. Using a gamma camera, the transport of bile to the gallbladder and the emptying of the gallbladder in response to a test meal can be visualized and quantified. The method is usually called HIDA (hepatic IDA) scintigraphy. Its use is limited.

2.8   Ultrasonography

Ultrasound can be used to visualize the filling and movements of some parts of the gastrointestinal canal. This can be done with an external probe, but also with a probe in the lumen of the gut.

External ultrasonography has been utilized to measure gallbladder volume and to study the emptying of the gallbladder after ingestion of a fatty meal or a chocolate bar (Fig. 2.15). The filling and emptying of the gallbladder in the fasting (interdigestive) state can also be studied with ultrasound.

Some centers use ultrasonography to assess gastric emptying. This can be done in two ways. First, one can measure the diameter of the gastric antrum at regular points in time after ingestion of a liquid meal. It has been shown that the decrease in antral diameter correlates well with the rate of gastric emptying. The second technique comprises

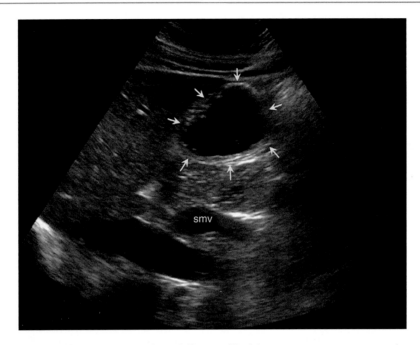

Fig. 2.15 Ultrasonographic measurement of antral diameter. Used in some centers to assess gastric emptying. The *arrows* point at the fluid-filled antrum (*smv* superior mesenteric vein)

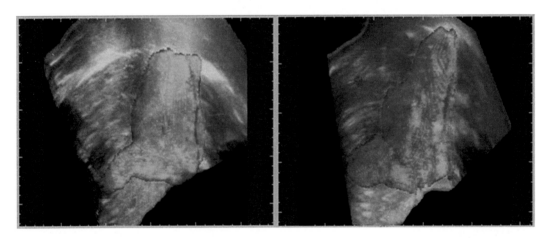

Fig. 2.16 Three-dimensional ultrasonography of the stomach. The reconstructed gastric volume is indicated in green. *Left panel*: stomach of healthy subject. *Right panel*: stomach of a patient with functional dyspepsia. In the patient with functional dyspepsia, a greater proportion of the meal is in the antrum, and a smaller proportion is in the corpus and fundus

three-dimensional reconstruction of the stomach based on a series of ultrasonographic images. From these three-dimensional images, the total gastric volume can be calculated, and gastric emptying can be quantified (Fig. 2.16).

So far, the endoscopic ultrasonographic assessment of movements of the gastrointestinal tract wall has remained limited to the scientific research domain. For instance, longitudinal contractions of the esophagus, which cannot be detected manometrically, have been studied using EUS. These studies have shown that longitudinal esophageal contractions may play a role in the generation of symptoms such as heartburn and chest pain.

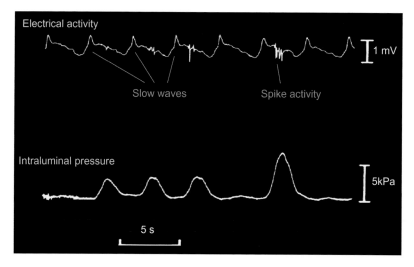

Fig. 2.17 Electrical (*upper tracing*) and mechanical activities (*lower tracing*) of the gastrointestinal tract. A continuous pattern of electrical slow waves can be seen. Slow waves with superimposed spike activity are associated with contractions, and slow waves without spikes are not

2.9   Electromyography

Not only striated but also smooth muscle generates electrical activity in association with contractions. Contraction-related electrical activity of smooth muscle cells usually takes the form of "spike potentials." In addition to these, muscle cells in the wall of the gastrointestinal canal also produce another type of electrical activity, which is also present when the cells are not mechanically active. This second type of electrical activity is called "basic electrical rhythm," "electrical control activity," or "slow waves" (Fig. 2.17). The frequency of the slow waves is different in each part of the tract. For instance, in humans, slow wave frequency in the stomach is 3/min, in the duodenum 12/min, and in the terminal ileum 7/min.

Electromyography of the smooth muscles of the gastrointestinal tract is a research technique; so far no clinical application has emerged yet. Electrodes can be brought in close proximity to the muscular layers from the mucosal (endoscopically) or from the serosal side (surgically). Using electromyography not only the slow waves but also the spike potentials can be recorded.

Electromyography of the striated muscles of the external anal sphincter and the pelvic floor can be carried out with needle electrodes that are inserted into these muscles or with surface electrodes. For electromyography of the external anal sphincter, a plug fitted with electrodes is inserted in the anal canal. In the past electromyography of the external anal sphincter has been used as a tool to localize a defect in the sphincter. Nowadays the preferred method for this purpose is anal ultrasonography.

2.10   Electrogastrography

Electrogastrography (EGG) is the technique that uses surface electrodes (placed on the skin) to measure the electrical activity generated by the smooth muscle layers of the stomach.

The electrogastrographic signal looks like a sine wave ("sinusoidal"). In man, the frequency of the signal is 2.8–3.2 cycles/min (Fig. 2.18). The signal can be recorded continuously, day and night, regardless of the presence of contractions in the distal stomach. When gastric contractions do occur, the amplitude of the sinusoidal EGG signal increases. Since the diagnostic value of EGG is extremely limited, the method is not in widespread use clinically.

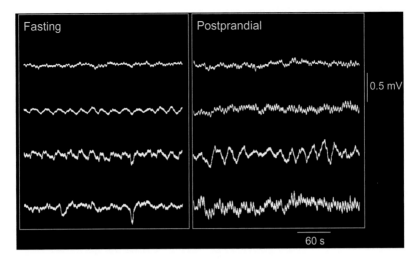

Fig. 2.18 Electrogastrographic signals recorded from a healthy subject. *Left panel*: fasting. *Right panel*: postprandial. After meal ingestion an increase in the amplitude of the sinusoid waves can be seen

2.11   Breath Tests

There are two different types of breath tests that can be used to obtain information on the rate of transit through the gastrointestinal tract. The first of these types is based on measurement of the concentration of hydrogen gas (H_2) in exhaled air after ingestion of a carbohydrate. The second type of test uses the nonradioactive carbon isotope ^{13}C to mark a test meal and measures the excretion of $^{13}CO_2$ in the exhaled air.

2.11.1 Hydrogen Breath Test

Hydrogen breath tests for measurement of orocecal transit time are based on the principle that bacteria in the colon can ferment undigested carbohydrates. In the process they produce hydrogen. The hydrogen gas is absorbed, at least in part, by the colon. Via the bloodstream, this gas reaches the lungs and there it is excreted in the expired air. When a test meal containing a nondigestible and nonabsorbable carbohydrate is ingested, this carbohydrate will reach the cecum unaltered. Depending on the composition of the meal, this will be the case after 90–120 min. Immediately after arrival of the carbohydrate in the colon, fermentation by bacteria starts, and hydrogen is produced as one of the breakdown products. The time interval between the ingestion of the test meal and the rise of the hydrogen concentration in the expired air reflects the mouth-to-cecum transit time (Fig. 2.19). One of the carbohydrates that is most often used for measurement of orocecal transit is the synthetic disaccharide lactulose. The test can also be carried with a meal rich in poorly absorbable carbohydrates in food items such as beans.

In the case of bacterial overgrowth of the small intestine, an unexpectedly early rise in the hydrogen concentration is seen, because bacteria in the small bowel start to metabolize the indigestible carbohydrates before they have reached the cecum. Understandably, it may be difficult to differentiate rapid orocecal transit from bacterial overgrowth.

2.11.2 ^{13}C Breath Test

Carbon-13 (^{13}C) is an isotope that is not radioactive. After ingestion of a meal labeled with this isotope, breakdown of the meal in the proximal small bowel will lead to the production of $^{13}CO_2$. After some time the $^{13}CO_2$ is excreted by the

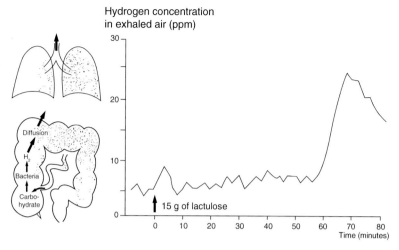

Fig. 2.19 Hydrogen breath test. After ingestion of 15 g of lactulose, the hydrogen concentration in the exhaled air increases as soon as the lactulose has reached the cecum

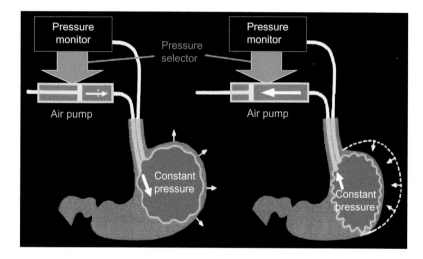

Fig. 2.20 Schematic representation of the barostat technique. An air pump keeps the pressure inside the intragastric bag constant. By continuously measuring the volume in the bag, gastric tone can be measured

lungs. The rate-limiting step in this cascade of events is the rate of gastric emptying. This makes it possible to measure gastric emptying by measuring the concentration of $^{13}CO_2$ repeatedly after ingestion of the isotope-labeled meal. The mathematical calculations required for this are rather complex. Often ^{13}C-octanoic acid is used to label the meal, because octanoic acid is not broken down in the stomach, absorbed in the proximal small bowel, and then metabolized. Gastric emptying is the rate-limiting step in this process of labeled CO_2 formation. The rate of gastric emptying as measured with the ^{13}C breath test correlates well with the rate measured with the gold standard technique, scintigraphy. The test is easy to perform and patient-friendly and finds widespread application.

2.11.3 Barostat Technique

The barostat is a specialized technique that was designed to measure tone in various parts of the gastrointestinal canal, in particular the proximal stomach and the colon. An air-filled bag made out of polyethylene is placed in the lumen. A dedicated air pump connected to the bag keeps the pressure in the bag constant. When the tone of the gut wall increases, the barostat pump sucks out air, to keep the pressure constant. Likewise, when the tone decreases, air is pumped into the bag (Fig. 2.20). The volume of air in the bag is continuously measured by the barostat device, and the changes in the intrabag volume reflect changes in tone. Because of the invasive and unpractical nature of the investigation,

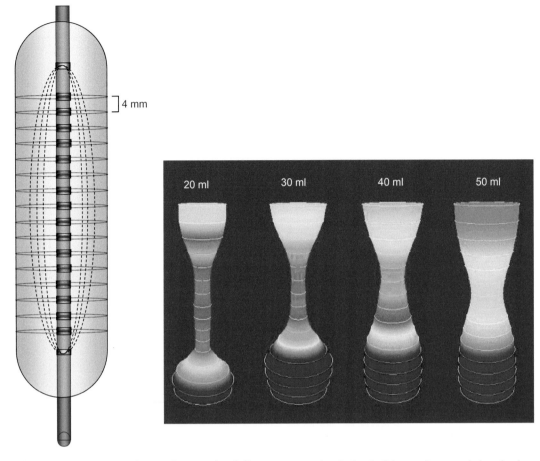

4 mm

Fig. 2.21 Impedance planimetry. Cross-sectional diameter is measured at 16 levels along the water-filled balloon. The four multicolor shapes represent diameters measured at the level of the esophagogastric junction in a healthy subject, with 20–50 ml water in the balloon

measurement of tone by the barostat is largely confined to the research domain.

The barostat can not only be used for measurement of tone but also for distension of parts of the gastrointestinal canal. The investigator can choose between volume- and pressure-controlled distension. Use of the barostat for distension most often occurs in research on the sensitivity of the gut (visceroperception). Some institutions use sensitivity testing as a diagnostic tool.

2.12   Impedance Planimetry

Impedance planimetry is a recent addition to the armamentarium of the motility lab. The system comprises a balloon catheter that measures cross-sectional area at 16 points along the length of the balloon using impedance planimetry. Sixteen electrodes mounted at close intervals on the shaft of the catheter inside the water-filled balloon measure the resistance for an alternative current. The impedance is proportional to cross-sectional area. Results are displayed in an intuitively interpretable two-dimensional topographical format (Fig. 2.21). By filling the balloon with increasing volumes of water, the distensibility of the surrounding tissue is tested. Using this technique it has been found that the distensibility of the esophagogastric junction is increased in patients with reflux disease and greatly decreased in patients with achalasia. The clinical relevance of impedance planimetry is not yet certain.

Principles of Drug Therapy for Disorders of Gastrointestinal Function

3

3.1 Introduction

The aim of diagnostic and physiological tests in patients with presumed disorders of gastrointestinal function is to establish a firm diagnosis, which allows specific treatment. However, the number of efficacious and specific treatment modalities for disorders of gastrointestinal function is limited. Very often, the treating physician has to resort to the usage of drugs that were developed for other conditions (off-label use), which may lead to confusion and can be implicated in the occurrence of adverse events. To date, no cure is available for disorders of gastrointestinal function. The therapeutic aim when dealing with disorders of gastrointestinal function is to alleviate the symptom burden associated with these conditions. Treatment approaches are directed either toward changing the contractility of the gastrointestinal tract, its secretory activity, or decreasing sensitivity (perception) of the gastrointestinal tract (Fig. 3.1).

3.2 Drugs That Enhance Contractility of the Gastrointestinal Tract

Whenever hypocontractility (too few contractions or contractions of too little force) is implicated in the pathogenesis of symptoms, treatments aimed at enhancing contractility can be used.

3.2.1 Direct Stimulation of Gastrointestinal Smooth Muscle

As the most important neurotransmitter involved in generating smooth muscle contraction in the gastrointestinal tract is acetylcholine, so-called cholinomimetic agents can be used. Examples are bethanechol, which mimics the activity of acetylcholine, or neostigmine, which inhibits the degradation of acetylcholine. The use of this class of agents induces direct stimulation of smooth muscle contractility, but this occurs in a non-organ-specific fashion, usually involving the whole gastrointestinal tract. Furthermore, this approach often generates poorly coordinated contractions (which lacks proper coordination of contractile and relaxant activities, as in the peristaltic reflex). Finally, this type of approach often also stimulates acetylcholine receptors outside of the gastrointestinal tract, including receptors on ocular musculature, salivary glands, and sweat glands. Consequently, at levels of effective stimulation of gastrointestinal contractions, adverse events due to non-gastrointestinal receptors often occur. For all of these reasons, the use of this class of agents is largely abandoned.

Tachykinins (including substance P) are a group of peptides that are often released together with acetylcholine, which generate strong contractions of smooth muscle cells. Agonists at tachykinin receptors seem less

© Springer International Publishing Switzerland 2016
A.J. Bredenoord et al., *A Guide to Gastrointestinal Motility Disorders*,
DOI 10.1007/978-3-319-26938-2_3

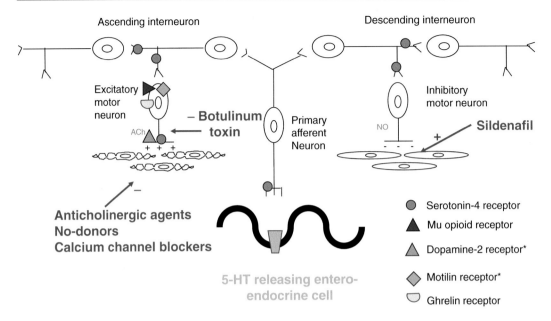

Fig. 3.1 Schematic overview of the control of gastrointestinal contractility through intrinsic neural pathways and potential targets for pharmacotherapy (*only in the proximal gastrointestinal tract: stomach and proximal small bowel)

suitable for treatment of disorders of gastrointestinal function due to the high likelihood of adverse events outside of the gastrointestinal tract (e.g., the respiratory system).

3.2.2 Stimulation of Contractions through Intrinsic Excitatory Nerves

Stimulation of nerves that control contractions is a more attractive target for stimulation of motility, as this is more likely to generate coordinated contractility. Several receptors that are expressed on intrinsic nerves of the gastrointestinal tract are a potential target for this approach. The serotonin-4 receptors, through which motility-enhancing drugs such as metoclopramide, cisapride, tegaserod, and prucalopride are acting, are an important target. They are expressed on nerve cells that generate and coordinate peristalsis and have been shown to enhance contractility from the esophagus to the colon and hence have seen application in gastroesophageal reflux disease, gastroparesis, and constipation.

Dopamine receptors are another suitable target for stimulating motility. Dopamine-2 receptors are mainly expressed in the stomach and the proximal small bowel. Stimulation of these receptors inhibits smooth muscle contractility, and antagonism of the receptors, through the action of drugs such as domperidone, enhances gastric and small bowel contractions. This can be used, for instance, in the treatment of gastroparesis. An additional advantage of this drug class is the involvement of the same dopamine-2 receptor in the generation of nausea and vomiting, and these symptoms can be controlled by dopamine-2 antagonists.

A third type of receptors that allows to enhance motility through stimulation of neural pathways is the motilin receptor, which is also mainly expressed in the stomach and the duodenum. Erythromycin, a well-known antibiotic, activates this receptor and thus stimulates gastric motility at doses which are far below those used for antibiotic purposes. Several variants of erythromycin, devoid of antibiotic properties and with strong stimulatory effects on gastric contractility, have been developed and studied, but the symptomatic benefit of these agents was limited, and to date, none has made it to the market.

Related to the motilin receptor is the ghrelin receptor. It is expressed on nerves in the stomach, the proximal small intestine, and the colon. A number of ghrelin receptor agonists are under evaluation for their ability to provide symptom benefit for disorders of gastrointestinal function.

3.3   Drugs That Inhibit Contractility of the Gastrointestinal Tract

When the presence of excessive contractions or a lack of muscle relaxation underlies symptoms, treatment can be advocated to inhibit contractility or enhance relaxation of smooth muscle.

3.3.1   Direct Inhibition of Smooth Muscle

Contractions of gastrointestinal smooth muscle require a rise of intracellular calcium. Hence, inhibition of calcium channels can be applied to inhibit contractility. This can be achieved through the use of L-type calcium channel blockers, such as nifedipine, amlodipine, or verapamil. However, these agents lack gastrointestinal specificity, and at doses that inhibit gastrointestinal contractility, often side effects occur due to vasodilation (such as low blood pressure, hot flushes, pounding headaches, and edema).

The so-called musculotropic spasmolytic agents, otilonium bromide, pinaverium bromide, and mebeverine, are a group of calcium channel blockers that act locally on the smooth muscle cells of the large intestine. They are used in the treatment of irritable bowel syndrome and, thanks to their local action, are well tolerated.

As nitric oxide (NO) is the most important neurotransmitter involved in inducing smooth muscle relaxation in the gastrointestinal tract, so-called NO-donors can also be used for pharmacotherapy of disorders of gastrointestinal function.

Examples are agents like isosorbide dinitrate or glyceryltrinitrate. The relaxant effect that these agents exert on smooth muscle is not organ specific, as they usually reach and influence the entire gastrointestinal tract. Furthermore, their administration may also affect smooth muscle cells in blood vessels, leading to adverse effects such as hypotension, hot flushes, pounding headaches, and edema.

Anticholinergics can also be used to inhibit contractions and thereby, indirectly, enhance inhibitory motor effects. The use of anticholinergics is associated with adverse effects outside the gastrointestinal tract (e.g., urinary retention, disturbances of ocular accommodation, dry mouth, etc.). Butylhyoscine bromide is an anticholinergic agent which, due to its quaternary ammonium structure, has limited systemic availability upon oral intake. It is often applied as short-term treatment in case of colic or crampy abdominal pain. Repeated administration is thought to lead to loss of efficacy. In addition, tricyclic antidepressants may also have some anticholinergic actions, which can be beneficial in the treatment of some disorders of gastrointestinal function (see below).

An approach which is related to NO is the use of phosphodiesterase inhibitors. The best-known agent in this class is sildenafil. This group of compounds, normally used for the treatment of erectile dysfunction, enhances the effect of NO on smooth muscle by prolonging the action of its second messenger cyclic guanosine monophosphate (GMP). This results in a relaxant effect on the gastrointestinal tract smooth muscle, although phosphodiesterase inhibitors are rarely used because of cost and vascular adverse effects.

3.3.2   Inhibition of Contractions through Intrinsic Inhibitory Nerves

Inhibition of contractions or stimulation of relaxation can also be achieved through neural pathways. Several receptors expressed on intrinsic nerves in the gastrointestinal tract are a potential target for this approach.

Local intramural injection of a low dose of botulinum toxin, which inhibits the release of acetylcholine for several months, is a relatively simple method to achieve a local relaxant effect. It is mainly applied in the lower esophageal sphincter (in achalasia), in the esophageal body (hypercontractility disorders), and in some other sphincters. A disadvantage is the need for retreatment when the toxin loses its effectiveness, which is usually after approximately 6 months.

Activation of opioid receptors on intrinsic nerves induces strong suppression of propulsive contractility. This underlies the well-known constipating effect of opioid analgesics. This is also applied therapeutically in the case of the peripherally acting (i.e., not in the brain) opioid agonist loperamide, which is used in the treatment of acute and chronic diarrhea. Meanwhile, peripherally acting opioid antagonists have also been developed (examples are methylnaltrexone and naloxegol) to counteract the constipating effects of opioid analgesics in the bowel, without loss of centrally mediated analgesic actions.

Somatostatin is the most important endogenous inhibitor of multiple gastrointestinal functions, including contractility. Somatostatin analogues, such as octreotide, pasireotide, and somatuline, have an inhibitory action on motility, but they are only available as injectable therapies because they are relatively large peptides. For this and for cost issues, these medications are used only sporadically in highly selected patients.

3.4   Medications That Change the Content of the Gastrointestinal Tract

Although the most logical approach in case of disorders of motility seems to target muscle cells and their innervation, changes in the content of the gastrointestinal lumen can also convey important, indirect, therapeutic effects. Moreover, many of these agents remain and act locally, which decreases the likelihood of important adverse effects.

3.4.1   Inhibition of Gastric Acid Secretion

Inhibition of the production of gastric acid is an important principle in the treatment of esophageal and gastric symptoms. For rapid relief of acid-related symptoms, antacids can be used, as they provide a rapid but short-lived neutralization of gastric acid. The most efficacious treatment is the use of proton pump inhibitors (such as omeprazole, lansoprazole, pantoprazole, rabeprazole, and esomeprazole), which directly inactivate the acid-secreting protein in the gastric parietal cells. They are most suitable for continuous daily usage. In case of gastroesophageal reflux disease and in a subset of functional dyspepsia patients, they generate symptom relief, and they are effective at healing esophageal lesions in reflux esophagitis (Fig. 3.2). For symptoms occurring less frequently, histamine-2 blockers (such as ranitidine, famotidine, or cimetidine) can be used, which are less potent but have a more rapid onset of action.

3.4.2   Stool Softeners

In case of constipation, a number of therapeutic agents act to soften consistency and increase volume of stool, based on two modes of action. First approach is the ingestion of nonabsorbable sugars (e.g., lactulose or lactitol) that undergo fermentation by colonic microbiota. This induces increased osmolality and attracts water to the stool which makes them softer and more voluminous. However, the bacterial fermentation may induce flatulence and bloating. Another approach is the intake of fiber or polyethylene glycol polymers. These molecules are not absorbed and act osmotically to attract water to the stools, making them softer and more voluminous. As nonabsorbable sugars and polyethylene polymers remain in the bowel lumen, they have little or no systemic side effects.

3.4.3   Intestinal Secretagogues

Intestinal secretagogues are substances that promote water secretion or inhibit water reabsorption

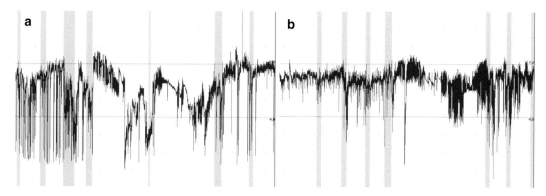

Fig. 3.2 A 24-h esophageal pH monitoring. The patient has interrupted the use of acid-suppressive medication 7 days prior to the first measurement, while acid-suppressive medication was continued during the second measurement. During the second measurement, the number of acid reflux episodes is considerably lower compared to the first one (142 reflux events without acid-suppressive therapy compared to 15 with acid-suppressive therapy). The lowest pH observed in the esophagus is higher during the second measurement compared to the first. There are still multiple pH drops during acid-suppressive therapy, but these drops are smaller and rarely reach levels below the pH threshold of 4. The acid exposure of the esophagus (time that esophageal pH is below 4) has decreased from 13.6 to 0.8 %

in the intestine, through luminal actions (Fig. 3.3). Lubiprostone is a lipophilic prostanoid compound, which acts locally to promote water and chloride secretion through activation of the CCl2 chloride channel on enterocytes. Doing so, it increases stool water content which softens stools and promotes propulsion. Linaclotide is an oligopeptide that acts as an agonist at the guanylate cyclase receptor on enterocytes. Activation of the receptor increases cyclic GMP levels in the enterocyte, which enhances chloride secretion through the cystic fibrosis transmembrane conductance regulator, also increasing stool water content. The stool-softening properties of lubiprostone and linaclotide are applied therapeutically in the treatment of constipation and irritable bowel syndrome with constipation.

3.4.4 Bile Salt Sequestration

The presence of bile salts in the large intestine is involved in the pathogenesis of worsening of some forms of diarrhea. Normally, bile salts are reabsorbed in the terminal ileum, but this process may be impaired in so-called bile salt malabsorption diarrhea or after surgery to the terminal ileum. Treatment with bile salt sequestrants, such as cholestyramine or colesevelam, is effective in these cases.

3.4.5 Alterations in the Intestinal Microbiome

The intestinal microflora plays a key role in the pathogenesis of diarrhea after antibiotic intake and may also be involved in symptom generation in some patients with the irritable bowel syndrome or with bloating, partly due to their fermenting metabolic activity. Pro- and prebiotic therapies are increasingly popular. Probiotic therapies aim at favorably altering intestinal microbiota through the ingestion of live bacteria, to provide symptom relief. In prebiotic therapies, the aim is to promote the growth of favorable microbes and inhibit the presence of less favorable ones, through ingestion of certain substances. Many different preparations are being studied, and many products, including some yoghurts and milks, are available that claim pro- or prebiotic effects. However, there is a paucity of consistent proof of efficacy, which seems to be limited and of lower magnitude than effects of drugs that are often used.

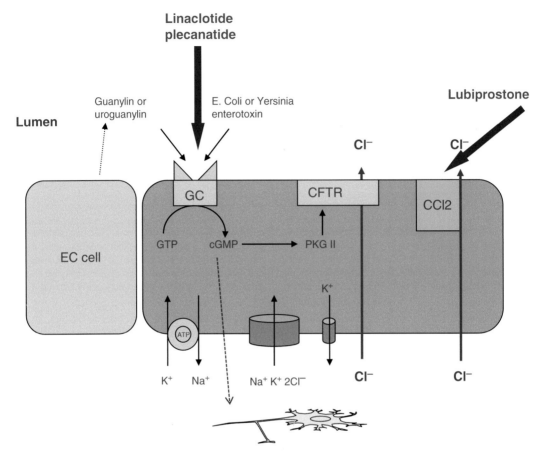

Fig. 3.3 Schematic overview of targets for enhancing intestinal secretion in the treatment of disorders with constipation. *EC* enterochromaffin, *GC* guanylate cyclase, *GTP* guanosine triphosphate, *cGMP* cyclic guanosine monophosphate, *CFTR* cystic fibrosis transmembrane conductance regulator, *CCl2* type 2 chloride channel

3.5 Medications That Alter the Sensitivity of the Gastrointestinal Tract

Although it seems logical to treat disorders of gastrointestinal motility with agents that alter contractility of the gastrointestinal tract, this approach is hampered by issues of efficacy and tolerance. Another approach is to decrease the sensitivity of the gastrointestinal tract, thereby suppressing signals that are generated by defective motor control or visceral hypersensitivity and thus decreasing symptom occurrence and severity.

No drugs are available that selectively decrease visceral sensitivity, but a number of observations suggest that antidepressants are able to decrease visceral sensitivity. For this reason, they can be used as second-line therapies for motility disorders that are difficult to control by conventional motility-modifying approaches. The high comorbidity levels of disorders of gastrointestinal function with anxiety or depression further support their use. Although antidepressants are often used in clinical practice, solid scientific proof of their efficacy has remained limited.

Older antidepressants (so-called tricyclic agents) also have a limited anticholinergic activity, which directs their use to disorders without constipation. As tricyclic antidepressant intake can be associated with sleepiness, they are generally administered in the evening. Newer antidepressants (serotonin and serotonin/noradrenaline reuptake inhibitors) lack anticholinergic effects and can stimulate intestinal transit. Hence, they are mainly used when there is no diarrhea. As they lack a sedative effect, they are usually administered in the morning.

In animal studies, guanylate cyclase agonists have acute visceral analgesic properties, mediated through actions of cyclic guanosine monophosphate on visceral afferents. The extent to which the same mechanism is active in man requires further studies.

The Esophagus

4

4.1 Anatomy of the Esophagus

The esophageal lining consists of multiple layers of squamous epithelium. The transition from esophageal to gastric mucosa is called the z-line, because of the z-shaped appearance that one can find during endoscopy (Fig. 4.1).

The muscular layers of the pharynx continuously pass into the muscles of the upper esophageal sphincter (UES); all are striated muscle fibers. The UES consists of bundles of the cricopharyngeal muscle, which proximally pass into bundles of the pharyngeal constrictor muscles and distally pass into bundles of the circular esophageal muscles. The UES is controlled by the same nerves as the pharyngeal muscles and stands under voluntary control.

The muscular wall of the esophagus consists of two layers, an inner circular muscle layer and an outer longitudinal muscle layer. The nervous network of the myenteric plexus is found between the two muscle layers. The proximal one third of the esophageal muscles is striated, the middle third is a transition from striated to smooth muscle, and the distal third consists entirely of smooth muscle.

The lower esophageal sphincter (LES) also consists of smooth muscle and can be regarded as a local specialization of the circular muscle layer. The LES is normally found at the level where the esophagus leaves the thorax and enters the abdomen through the diaphragmatic hiatus. The LES and the muscular fibers of the diaphragm together form a functional entity that serves as a protection against gastroesophageal reflux.

4.2 Swallowing and Esophageal Peristalsis

The first step of digestion takes place in the mouth. By chewing, food is grinded and mixed with saliva. Saliva serves as a lubricant and contains amylase, an enzyme that digests starch. The muscles of the mouth and tongue push the food to the throat so it can be swallowed. In resting state, the esophagus is empty and the lumen is collapsed. The UES and LES exert a tonic pressure and seal off the esophagus. The onset of a swallow is voluntary, but the rest of the sequence that follows is reflexogenic. Swallowing is a well-organized movement of the mouth, tongue, throat, esophagus, and sphincters and results in transport of a bolus from the mouth to stomach. The swallow reflex inhibits respiration temporarily so that food does not enter the airways during swallowing. The swallow reflex starts when pressure sensors in the pharynx are stimulated. This activates an afferent nerve to the swallow center in brainstem. From there, motor neurons of the cranial nerves are activated that control the muscles of pharynx and upper esophagus (glossopharyngeal, vagal, and hypoglossal nerves) and the motor neurons of the vagus nerve that control the middle and distal esophagus.

© Springer International Publishing Switzerland 2016
A.J. Bredenoord et al., *A Guide to Gastrointestinal Motility Disorders*,
DOI 10.1007/978-3-319-26938-2_4

Fig. 4.1 Schematic display of the anatomy of the esophagus (Published with kind permission of © Rogier Trompert Medical Art 2015)

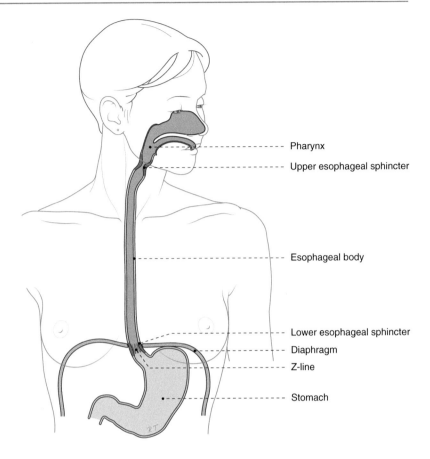

Pharynx

Upper esophageal sphincter

Esophageal body

Lower esophageal sphincter

Diaphragm

Z-line

Stomach

A swallow can be divided into three phases, which are the oral phase, the pharyngeal phase, and the esophageal phase. In the oral phase the swallow is still under voluntary control. This phase starts when the tongue pushes part of the food in the mouth against the palate and moves it toward the back of the mouth. When the bolus reaches the pharynx, the pressure sensors will be activated and the swallow reflex will start.

The pharyngeal phase is entirely reflexogenic and consists of the following steps:

1. The soft palate moves upward caused by the bolus below and closes off the nasopharynx.
2. The vocal cords close and the larynx moves upward against the epiglottis. This prevents the bolus from entering into the airways and facilitates opening of the UES.
3. The UES relaxes and the pharyngeal constrictors contract so the bolus is moved in distal direction.

4. A peristaltic wave starts above the pharynx and moves in distal direction. This will push the bolus through the relaxed UES.

The bolus has entered the esophagus and the esophageal swallow phase has been initiated. After the bolus has passed the UES, the sphincter will close. The peristaltic wave initiated by the swallow (primary peristalsis) moves further in distal direction with a propagating velocity of 3–5 cm/s. The peristaltic wave will have traversed the esophagus in about 10 s. Peristalsis ensures that passage of food is also possible in supine position; gravity thus only plays a minor role.

If the esophagus is dilated in the absence of a swallowing, for example, during inflation of air during endoscopy, peristalsis will be triggered. This is called secondary peristalsis. The peristaltic wave will then start at the position where the distention took place.

The volume and viscosity of the bolus influence the amplitude and velocity of propagation of the peristaltic wave via input of sensory nerves to the enteric nervous system and central nervous system.

During swallowing the LES relaxes so the bolus can pass the sphincter and reach the stomach. After relaxation the sphincter contracts and returns to the tonic pressure of approximately 20 mmHg.

A swallowed liquid bolus usually passes the esophagus in one swallow, for a solid bolus temporarily hold-up halfway in the esophagus is not uncommon and only after several swallows the bolus is cleared from the esophagus.

4.3   Belches

With every swallow, some air is introduced into the esophagus. This air is transported to the stomach, together with the swallowed bolus. Gas can also be formed in the stomach, for example, after drinking carbon dioxide-containing beverages. In upright position the gas will move to the proximal stomach. Stretching of the fundus by the gas will activate stretch sensors in the gastric wall, and through afferent fibers of the vagal nerve, a reflex is initiated that results in relaxation of the LES so that the air can escape the stomach. The relaxation of the LES is in this case not triggered by a swallow and is called transient LES relaxation (TLESR). This reflex prevents overdistention of the stomach. When the air reaches the esophagus, it can either trigger secondary peristalsis and being pushed back to the stomach or, when the air reaches the proximal esophagus, it can induce reflexogenic relaxation of the UES and the air can escape. The vibrations of the pharyngeal structures caused by the air passage cause the typical sound associated with belching.

4.4   Motility Disorders of the Esophagus

Disorders of motility of the esophagus can lead to ineffective transport of food from the mouth to the stomach. This can cause difficulty in swallowing, the feeling of impaired esophageal bolus transit and retrosternal pain. When there is a sensation of difficulty in propulsion of food from the mouth or throat to the esophagus, it is called oropharyngeal dysphagia. When there is a sensation of the food not further passing down through the esophagus, it is called esophageal dysphagia. Pain can be caused by a bolus that gets stuck and stretches the esophageal wall or because spastic contractions are induced. This symptom is also known as odynophagia. Of course, dysphagia can also be caused by narrowing of the esophagus, such as occurs with a tumor or peptic stricture after long-standing reflux disease. In case of esophageal motility disorders, there is often esophageal dysphagia for both solid and liquid foods, while in case of obstructive disorders, there is often dysphagia for solids only.

Esophageal motility disorders are classified into primary and secondary motility disorders. Secondary motility disorders are caused by another disease, for example, scleroderma that affects the esophageal muscles.

In case of esophageal dysphagia, the first step is to exclude an organic cause using endoscopy. Biopsies are always taken to exclude the presence of allergic or eosinophilic esophagitis, even when the esophagus has a normal endoscopic appearance. When endoscopy did not reveal any abnormalities and biopsies are normal, further testing for motility disorders will be performed. Usually, the next step is esophageal manometry (Fig. 4.2). A barium esophagogram is made when there is a suspicion for a stricture (Fig. 4.3).

4.5   Primary Esophageal Motility Disorders

4.5.1   Oropharyngeal Dysphagia

Dyskinesia of the UES is defined as a condition with poorly coordinated movements of the hypopharynx and UES. This results in symptoms of swallowing difficulty or aspiration. The sphincter may relax too late, too early, or not enough. Cricopharyngeal hypertrophy may also cause

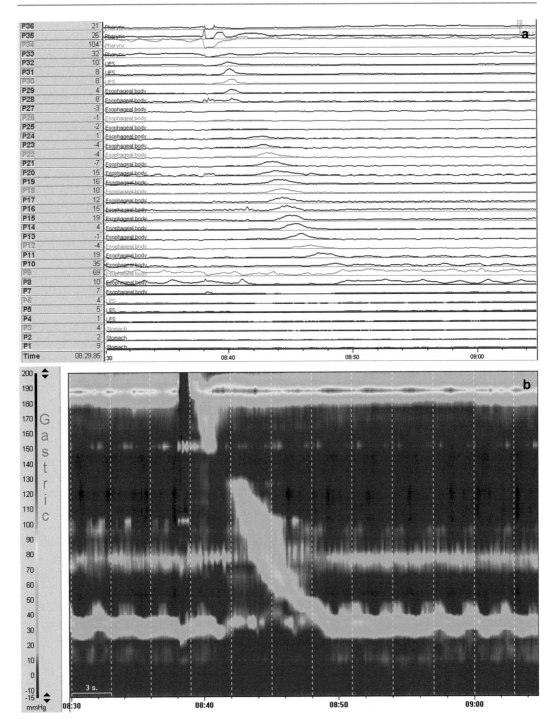

Fig. 4.2 Esophageal manometry in a subject with normal esophageal motility. Both conventional line tracings (**a**) are shown as well as colorplot tracings (**b**) as used in high-resolution manometry

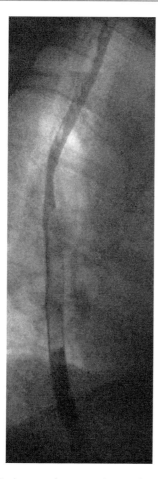

Fig. 4.3 Barium esophagogram in a patient with mid-esophageal narrowing of lumen caused by eosinophilic esophagitis

swallowing difficulties and aspiration. In this condition the resting pressure of the UES is increased and a Zenker's diverticulum is formed just above the sphincter.

Because the first phase of swallowing is controlled by the central nervous system through the cranial nerves, disorders of the central nervous system and cranial nerves such as tumors, neurodegenerative disorders, and stroke also result in swallowing disorders. For example, swallowing disorders are highly frequent in Parkinson's disease, sometimes making oral feeding impossible.

4.5.2 Esophageal Dysphagia

4.5.2.1 Achalasia

Achalasia is a disorder characterized by incomplete or absent relaxation of LES, in combination with absent esophageal peristalsis.

The severe abnormalities in esophageal motility are caused by destruction of the myenteric plexus. The cause for this is unknown but there are several hypotheses. It has been suggested that achalasia is partly genetic, an autoimmune disease, or caused by a virus. Achalasia can also be secondary to Chagas' disease; in that case the ganglia are destroyed by the parasite *Trypanosoma cruzi*, which lives only in South America.

Achalasia can have its first presentation in patients of all ages, equally frequent in men and women. It may take long before a diagnosis is made, because the disease is rare and unknown and because the disease often starts slowly. The final diagnosis is made with esophageal manometry.

The symptoms in achalasia are caused by the inability of the esophagus to empty. This results in problems with food passage; swallowed foods may stick in the esophagus for hours before they are regurgitated again. Retrosternal pain can be caused by stretch on the walls of the esophagus, due to stasis of food, but probably also by spastic contractions. Weight loss is also common. Longstanding achalasia can result in dilatation of the esophageal body (Fig. 4.4).

High-resolution manometry has revealed that there are several achalasia subtypes (Fig. 4.5). We distinguish classic achalasia (type I), achalasia with simultaneous increases in esophageal luminal pressure called pan-esophageal pressurization (type II), and achalasia with spastic contractions (type III). The achalasia subtypes differ in presentation, findings on manometry and barium esophagograms, and response to treatment.

The treatment of achalasia is focused on reduction of LES pressure, and this can be done in several ways. Medication such as nitrates and calcium channel blockers are insufficiently effective for long-term achalasia treatment. Botulinum

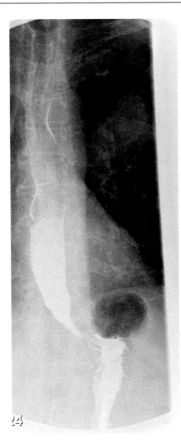

Fig. 4.4 Barium swallow radiograph in a patient with achalasia. The esophageal lumen is distended, while at the level of the transition from the esophagus to the stomach, there is hardly any contrast visible (bird's beak)

Surgical treatment consists of a laparoscopic cleavage of the LES, myotomy according Heller. Usually this procedure is combined with a fundoplication according to Dor to reduce any reflux after the myotomy. Reflux symptoms may occur after all successful treatments for achalasia, as the sphincter pressure will be reduced and there is no peristalsis in the esophagus to clear refluxed gastric contents. Heller myotomy is very effective and 80–90 % of the patients treated will not need future re-treatments. However, the treatment is more invasive than endoscopic treatments and complications such as esophageal mucosal perforations do occur.

Recently, it has also become possible to perform a myotomy using an endoscopic approach. In a so-called per-oral endoscopic myotomy (POEM) procedure, the LES is cut endoscopically. The procedure is promising but it is new and long-term results are not available yet.

Esophagogastric junction outflow obstruction is a disorder characterized by poor relaxation of the LES in combination with sufficient evidence of esophageal peristalsis. Typical symptoms are chest pain and dysphagia and the disorder may be an early stage of achalasia. Not all patients with manometric signs of esophagogastric junction outflow obstruction need treatment; symptoms may disappear spontaneously.

toxin (Botox) can be injected endoscopically at the level of the LES. This is an effective and relatively safe treatment option that is mostly performed under mild sedation. Disadvantage is that the effect wears out after 3–6 months and frequent retreatment will be required.

Pneumodilation is another treatment option. A 3- to 4-cm wide balloon is placed endoscopically or under fluoroscopic control at the level of the LES. By filling the balloon with air (pneumodilation), the sphincter is dilated. The effect of pneumodilation persists longer than that of Botox injections, but sometimes repeated dilations are required. There is also a risk of perforation of the esophagus (about 2 %). With repeat dilations when indicated, long-term symptom control can be achieved in 70–90 % of patients.

4.5.2.2 Distal Esophageal Spasm

Spastic contractions of esophageal muscles can cause retrosternal pain and dysphagia. Sometimes these pains come in attacks and may mimic cardiac pain. Not infrequently patients have been admitted to a coronary care unit several times before they are referred to the gastroenterologist for analysis of their noncardiac chest pain. Distal esophageal spasms are diagnosed with esophageal manometry (Fig. 4.6). Premature rapid propagating contractions are seen in the esophagus. Sometimes spastic contractions are also seen during endoscopy and on radiographic images (Fig. 4.7).

Attacks of spasms are frequently triggered by emotions or by eating food. Gastroesophageal reflux can also trigger spasms. Sometimes patients have symptom very infrequently, which

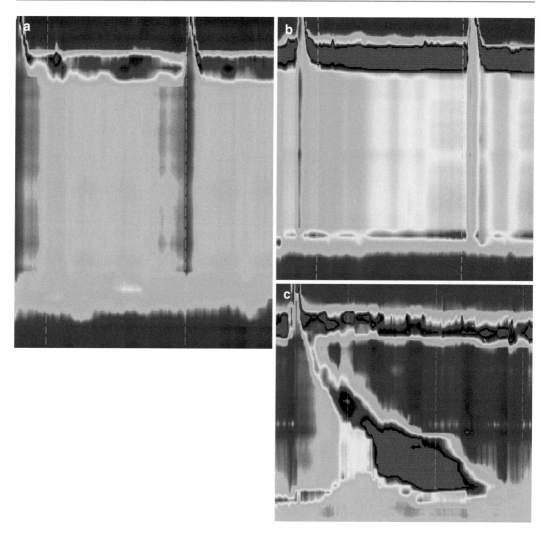

Fig. 4.5 High-resolution manometry of achalasia subtypes. Type I achalasia (**a**) shows limited pan-esophageal pressurization after swallows; in the type II achalasia (**b**) there is pronounced pan-esophageal pressurization visible. Type III achalasia (**c**) is characterized by spastic contractions

can make it difficult to make a diagnosis as the spastic contractions may not be visible on manometry in asymptomatic periods.

For management of spasms, it is of utmost importance to explain about the cause of the pain. Once the patients understand that the pain is caused by a benign disorder, this will substantially reduce anxiety during an attack. Medications that induce smooth muscle relaxation, such as nitroglycerine and calcium channel blockers, are moderately effective, although side effects such as headaches and hypotension may complicate effective dosing. In case of severe symptoms and insufficient effect of medication, endoscopic injections with botulinum toxin or even myotomy may be considered. Of course, when there is suspicion that reflux plays a role, this will need to be treated as well. Generally, the vast majority of patients with spasms use acid suppressants.

4.5.2.3 Hypercontractile Esophagus
The diagnosis hypercontractile esophagus is made when the contraction amplitude (or distal contraction integral) is abnormally high, while there is normal esophagogastric junction relaxation

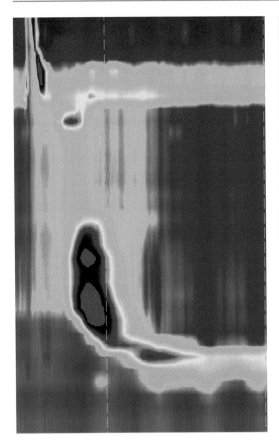

Fig. 4.6 High-resolution manometry picture of spastic contraction in distal esophagus

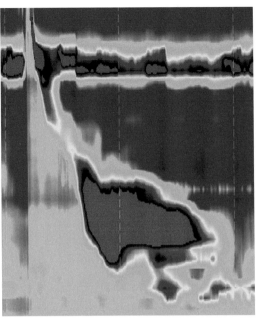

Fig. 4.8 High-resolution manometry showing a Jackhammer esophagus motility pattern with very strong contraction in the distal esophageal body but normal LES relaxation

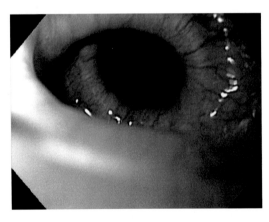

Fig. 4.7 Endoscopic picture of spastic contractions in the esophagus

(Fig. 4.8). In the era of conventional manometry, this was sometimes called nutcracker esophagus. In some cases the contraction wave is also often abnormally long, repetitive or multi-peaked; hence this condition is sometimes referred to as jackhammer esophagus. Sometimes, the condition may appear spastic. Hypercontractile esophagus is associated with symptoms of chest pain and dysphagia and treatment is similar to the treatment of distal esophageal spasms. Similar to spasm, reflux can play a role.

Absent Contractility

When there are no signs of peristaltic contractions but the LES relaxation is normal, the condition is characterized as absent contractility or sometimes called aperistalsis. This condition clearly differs from achalasia, and a barium swallow in patients with absent peristalsis typically reveals normal passage over the LES. Absent contractility can be asymptomatic or can be associated with dysphagia. It is sometimes seen secondary to systemic sclerosis. There is no effective treatment for absent contractility. When concurrent reflux disease is present, this is treated medically as antireflux surgery is considered contraindicated in patients with absent peristalsis.

4.5.2.4 Minor Disorders of Peristalsis

Ineffective esophageal motility and fragmented peristalsis are so-called minor disorders of peristalsis. Ineffective esophageal motility is characterized by a very low amplitude of the peristaltic contractions. Fragmented peristalsis is characterized by the presence of large pressure breaks in the peristaltic contractions in the esophagus. These disorders are often seen in patients with reflux disease. On one end weak contractions impair clearance of refluxed gastric contents; on the other end chronic excessive acid exposure leads to weakening of peristaltic function. Treatment with acid-suppressing medication will sometimes lead to improvement in esophageal motility as well. Prokinetic drugs have no established efficacy for improvement of esophageal hypocontractility. Minor disorders of peristalsis are not considered a contraindication for antireflux surgery. Long-term follow-up of the minor disorders of peristalsis is favorable, showing little to no progression to major motility disorders.

4.6   Secondary Esophageal Motility Disorders

Sometimes the esophageal motility disorder is the result of another disease; it is then called a secondary motility disorder. In patients with scleroderma, CREST (calcinosis, Raynaud phenomenon, esophageal motility disorder, sclerodactyly, telangiectasia), and mixed connective tissue disease, the smooth muscles of the esophagus can be involved, causing very weak to absent peristalsis in the distal esophagus. The pressure in the LES is usually also very low. In cases of polymyositis and dermatomyositis, the striated muscles of the esophagus can be involved. Usually, patients develop oropharyngeal dysphagia and frequent aspiration is possible. The proximal esophagus can also be involved in diseases that result in muscular atrophy of striated muscles. More rarely esophageal motility is involved in neuropathic diseases, diabetic mellitus, and CIIP (chronic idiopathic intestinal pseudo-obstruction).

4.7   Gastroesophageal Reflux Disease

Gastroesophageal reflux is a physiological phenomenon and occurs in healthy subjects approximately twenty times a day. In these subjects reflux is called physiological because it does not cause any damage and it occurs unnoticed without causing any symptoms. Reflux becomes gastroesophageal reflux disease (GERD) when it causes mucosal damage or bothersome symptoms (Fig. 4.9). In resting state the LES is closed and together with the right crus of the diaphragm forms a tight barrier against reflux of gastric contents.

We distinguish typical reflux symptoms and atypical reflux symptoms. Heartburn and regurgitation are considered typical reflux symptoms; chest pain, cough, hoarseness, and wheezing are considered atypical reflux symptoms. For atypical reflux symptoms, the relationship with reflux is often much less clear. Reflux can also cause dental erosions and laryngitis. When reflux causes symptoms proximal of the esophagus, it is often referred to as supra-esophageal reflux disease.

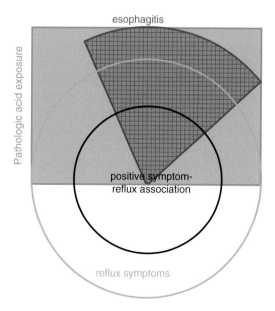

Fig. 4.9 Relationship between esophagitis, symptoms, and esophageal acid exposure. These entities are clearly related, but not the same

4.8   Pathophysiology of GERD

Two factors play an important role in GERD. Reflux of gastric contents can occur too frequently or in too large volumes, causing symptoms and mucosal damage. But the esophagus can also become hypersensitive to the presence of reflux; this leads to symptoms as well. In GERD patients a combination of both excessive reflux and hypersensitivity is often present. Reflux is considered excessive when there are more than 75 reflux episodes per day (50 acid reflux episodes per day) or when the esophagus is acidic (pH lower than 4) for more than 6 % of the time. These values are based on the upper limit of normal, measured as the 95th percentile in healthy subjects. The quantity of reflux is the resultant of the balance between defense against reflux and factors that promote reflux.

4.8.1   Defense Against Reflux

4.8.1.1 The Antireflux Barrier

Under normal conditions, the pressure in the abdominal compartment is higher than the pressure in the thoracic compartment. Therefore a firm barrier is required in order to prevent gastric content flow into the esophagus. The antireflux barrier consists of the LES and the right crus of the diaphragm. In resting conditions the LES is closed and exerts a tonic pressure, so it prevents retrograde flow of gastric contents over the LES. The diaphragm exerts little pressure to the antireflux barrier in the resting state. During activities that increase intra-abdominal pressure, such as deep inspiration, coughing, and bending over, the diaphragm contracts at the same time, resulting in a simultaneous increase in sphincter pressure. This prevents reflux during these activities.

The resting pressure of the LES varies during the day and is dependent on several factors:

- After the meal the sphincter pressure is lower than in fasted state. The sphincter pressure is mainly decreased by fatty meals, but also smoking and alcohol intake decrease sphincter pressure.
- In the phase of the migrating motor complex (MMC), the highest sphincter pressure is found during phase 3 and the lowest pressure during phase 1.
- Hormones. Progesterone decreases sphincter pressure, resulting in more reflux during pregnancy (in adjunction to a higher abdominal pressure).
- Medications. Several drugs decrease sphincter pressure.

The sphincter pressure thus varies and the relationship between sphincter pressure and the occurrence of reflux is only weak. Sphincter pressure mainly plays an important role when it is so low that the sphincter barely forms an effective barrier anymore.

Most reflux occurs during the so-called transient LES relaxations (TLESRs). TLESRs are relaxations that are not triggered by a swallow but instead are induced by stretch of the wall of the gastric fundus induced by accumulation of swallowed air or ingested food or liquids. These TLESRs are part of the physiological venting mechanism of the stomach, allowing air to escape. However, TLESRs also allow reflux of liquid gastric content. TLESRs are not more frequent in patients with GERD than in others, but TLESRs in GERD patients are more often accompanied with liquid reflux of gastric contents.

4.8.1.2 Clearance of Reflux

As mentioned before, reflux is physiological and occurs in every human. The duration of the presence of refluxed gastric content in the esophagus depends on the clearance. Volume clearance and chemical clearance are distinguished. Sudden filling of the esophagus with reflux from the stomach results in stretch of the esophageal wall and subsequent secondary peristalsis. The peristaltic wave will push most of the refluxed liquids back to the stomach. A thin layer of noxious acidic gastric liquids will remain on the esophageal wall. This acid film will gradually be neutralized by swallowed alkaline saliva. This explains why nocturnal reflux remains much longer in the esophagus. Indeed during sleep there is reduced saliva production and a lower swallowing frequency which leads to a slower volume and chemical clearance.

4.8.2 Factors Promoting Reflux

4.8.2.1 Hiatus Hernia

In case of a hiatus hernia, the LES is migrated a few centimeters in oral direction and is not at the same level as the diaphragm anymore. This occurs when the ligaments keeping the distal esophagus at its place become looser. The consequence is that the most proximal part of the stomach is located above the diaphragm, in the thoracic compartment (Fig. 4.10).

A hiatus hernia results in a serious weakening of the antireflux barrier because the synergy between the diaphragm and LES has ceased. The hernia bag can also function as a reservoir of gastric acid, from which reflux occurs with every relaxation of the LES, thus with each swallow. The size of a hernia varies constantly

and the distal esophagus can slide through the diaphragmatic opening (sliding hernia). This is the reason why a hernia can be missed during endoscopy.

4.8.2.2 Obesity

In obese patients the pressure in the abdominal compartment is increased, which leads to a more substantial pressure gradient from the stomach to the esophagus and facilitates reflux. In addition to this, most obese patients have a hiatus hernia, which makes the antireflux barrier weaker. Obesity is thus a risk factor for reflux disease.

4.8.2.3 Large Meals

Most reflux episodes occur in the postprandial period. The filling of the stomach reduces sphincter pressure and triggers more TLESRs. Also, the acid production is stimulated by the presence of foods. Furthermore, a meal leads to floating of an acid layer on top of the food, the so-called acid pocket, which serves as a reservoir

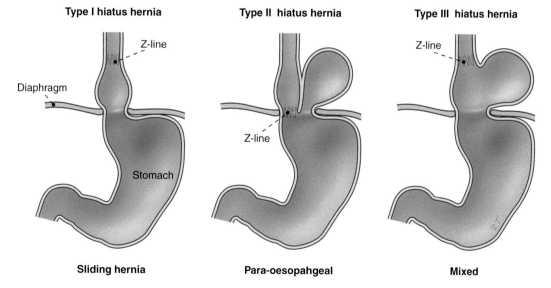

Fig. 4.10 Different types of hernias. In case of a sliding hernia, a part of the proximal stomach is located above the diaphragm; above it is the esophagus. The herniated part of the stomach slides through the diaphragmatic opening; hence it is called sliding hernia. Part of the time the hernia is present, part of the time the hernia is reduced, and the LES and diaphragm are located at the same level. This makes that a hernia can be missed with examinations such as endoscopy or barium swallow. Also in case of a parae-sophageal hernia, part of the proximal stomach is located above the diaphragm, but in this type of hernia the esophagus is located next to it and not above it. A type III hernia or mixed-type hernia is a combination of both a sliding and paraesophageal hernia (Published with kind permission of © Rogier Trompert Medical Art 2015)

for acid reflux. A large meal thus increases the number of reflux episodes.

4.8.2.4 Delayed Gastric Emptying

A delayed gastric emptying usually only plays a small role in the pathogenesis of reflux disease. Only in case of severe gastric emptying disturbances or gastroparesis an important increase in reflux is found, because the postprandial phase – with filled stomach – lasts longer.

4.8.2.5 The Constituents of Reflux

In most patients with GERD, the constituents of gastric contents and of reflux are not different from those found in healthy subjects. Increased acid production is not an issue in GERD; the problem is acid moving in the wrong direction. The acidity of the stomach is usually well below pH 4. During a meal the gastric contents are buffered and the pH increases temporarily, after which the pH is decreased again due to increased acid production. Reflux is thus generally acidic. In addition to acid, gastric juice also contains the enzyme pepsin which breaks down proteins. Sometimes reflux also contains bile acids and bilirubin that are refluxed from the small bowel into the stomach. This is of course more frequent when the pyloric sphincter is not intact anymore, such as occurs after a Billroth II partial gastric resection. Immediately after a meal, when the gastric contents are buffered, most reflux episodes are not so acidic. Reflux is called weakly acidic when the pH lies between 4 and 7. Sometimes the pH of reflux is even higher than 7; this is called weakly alkaline reflux. Weakly alkaline reflux is not synonymous with bile reflux; acid reflux can also contain bile acids.

4.8.3   Hypersensitivity of the Esophagus

A pathologically high exposure of the esophagus to reflux of gastric contents not necessarily leads to reflux symptoms. On the other hand, patients with reflux symptoms can have a normal quantity of reflux. Damage of the esophageal mucosa can lead to enhanced sensitivity of the esophagus, but also a macroscopically normal esophagus can

sense reflux. Exposure to acid seems to enhance the sensitivity of the esophagus to subsequent reflux episodes. In addition to that, the sensitivity of the esophagus is increased during periods with increased psychological stress.

4.8.4   Reflux Esophagitis

The gastric mucosa is highly resistant to gastric acid and pepsin; the esophageal mucosa however lacks such resistance. The esophagus can be severely damaged by reflux. The distal esophagus is most often affected; this is the part with most contact to gastric acid. Damage of the esophagus by reflux leads to specific erosive lesions called reflux esophagitis. Reflux esophagitis is a reversible disorder that usually heals during acid suppressant treatment. However, when the esophagus is frequently exposed to gastric acid and especially when the exposure is prolonged, scarring with stricture formation can occur (Fig. 4.11). A significant peptic stricture results in dysphagia for solid foods.

Long-standing reflux can also result in metaplasia of the esophageal mucosa. The epithelium will acquire characteristics of small bowel mucosa instead of its normal multilayer squamous mucosa. This is called Barrett mucosa. Barrett mucosa can become dysplastic, which means its characteristics change and it becomes a risk factor for development

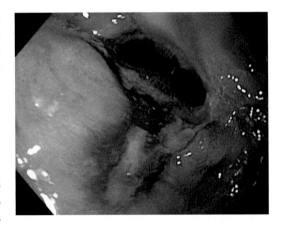

Fig. 4.11 Endoscopic image of a peptic stricture at the level of the esophagogastric junction. The pale tissue is fibrous tissue that has led to significant structuring of the distal esophagus. A peptic stricture can be dilated with a balloon or bougie

of esophageal adenocarcinoma. In subjects with Barrett mucosa, the chance of developing an adenocarcinoma of the esophagus is significantly increased, which is why Barrett mucosa is regarded a premalignant condition. Periodical endoscopic surveillance with biopsies is therefore recommended in patients with proven Barrett mucosa.

4.9   Diagnosis of Gastroesophageal Reflux Disease

Gastroesophageal reflux disease is present when there is either damage to the esophageal mucosa as a result of gastroesophageal reflux or when reflux results in bothersome symptoms. The diagnosis of GERD is thus established when mucosal damage is demonstrated or when it is proven that patient's symptoms are related to reflux. A single test that can demonstrate both does not exist. Mucosal damage is usually observed with endoscopy, while ambulatory reflux monitoring can demonstrate whether there is a relationship between patient's symptoms and reflux. History alone is not reliable for making the diagnosis of GERD; symptoms are neither specific nor sensitive for GERD.

4.9.1   PPI Test

A PPI test is short treatment period with a PPI, usually 14 days. When there is a significant decrease (>50 %) in symptoms during this treatment period, the test is considered to be positive. However, a symptomatic response to acid secretion inhibition is not only seen in patients with GERD but also in other patients such as those with peptic ulcer disease and functional dyspepsia. A placebo effect can also play an important role in symptom reduction, and thus, the specificity of the test is low. Furthermore, absence of response can be seen in GERD patients with symptoms due to weakly acidic reflux. The PPI test is mainly popular in primary care and is attractive when absolute diagnostic certainty is not required. For secondary care, the PPI test is not appropriate.

4.9.2   Endoscopy

Endoscopy is the most used diagnostic test to detect the presence of GERD and rule out other disorders in secondary care. Typical reflux esophagitis proves the presence of GERD, and with endoscopy the severity of mucosal damage can be determined. This is expressed using the Los Angeles classification (Fig. 4.12).

Endoscopy also allows detection of complications of GERD, such as a peptic stricture, a Schatzki ring, and Barrett mucosa (Fig. 4.13). The presence of hiatus hernia is a risk factor for GERD but has no diagnostic value. An irregular z-line and an erythematous mucosa suggest a high esophageal acid exposure of the mucosa but also are not specific for GERD and do not prove that a patient's symptoms are due to reflux.

In most patients with reflux symptoms, no abnormalities are detected during endoscopy.

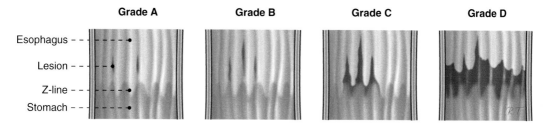

Fig. 4.12 Schematic representation of the Los Angeles classification of reflux esophagitis. In Los Angeles grade A, there are mucosal lesions of maximally 5 mm in length. In grade B the lesion is more than 5 mm in length. In grade C the mucosal lesion extends between two folds and thus connects the lesions on top of the folds. The damaged mucosa involves less than 75 % of the circumference. In grade D the mucosal lesions involves more than 75 % of the esophageal circumference (Published with kind permission of © Rogier Trompert Medical Art 2015)

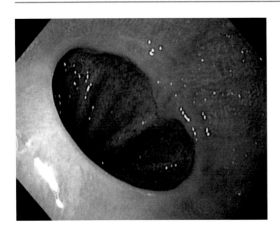

Fig. 4.13 Endoscopic image of a Schatzki ring. A Schatzki ring is a relative stricture at the level of the *z*-line in patients with a hiatus hernia. Although mostly asymptomatic, large pieces of solid food can get stuck proximal to the narrowing (Published with kind permission of © Rogier Trompert Medical Art 2015)

This is partly due to the fact that most patients will use acid suppressant medication during endoscopy, which will already have healed most lesions. The absence of mucosal lesions therefore does not exclude GERD. Although the specificity of endoscopy for the diagnosis of GERD is high, it is not a very sensitive method to diagnose GERD. Taking esophageal biopsies during endoscopy is not routinely recommended. There are certainly microscopic abnormalities associated with GERD, but these have no diagnostic value. This does not exclude that, for example, in case of dysphagia or recurrent food impactions, biopsy taking is required when other disorders such as eosinophilic esophagitis are in the differential.

4.9.3   Ambulatory Reflux Monitoring

Ambulatory pH monitoring allows prolonged measurement of acid exposure in the esophagus, usually during 24 h (Fig. 4.14). Through the nose a catheter is placed in the esophagus of the patient. The catheter is connected to a data recorder which stores the data. The patient usually returns the next day and the data are downloaded from the data recorder. During the measurement, patients will indicate when they perceive any symptoms using the event marker button. Afterwards, it is analyzed whether symptoms were preceded by reflux events. This allows conclusions on whether or not symptoms are reflux related or not. The relationship between symptoms and reflux episodes are usually expressed using symptom-reflux association indices, such as the symptom index (SI) and the symptom association probability (SAP) (Fig. 4.15).

Ambulatory reflux monitoring can also be performed using a wireless pH detection device, which is attached to the esophageal wall. Attachment of the pH sensor is usually guided endoscopically. The sensor will transmit its signals to a data recorder outside the patient. The advantage of wireless pH measurement is that it causes much less discomfort compared to the naso-esophageal catheters. This allows extension of the measurement duration to 48 and even 72 h. The most important disadvantage of the technique is the relatively high cost.

A normal, physiological acid exposure in the esophagus does not rule out GERD. It is possible that patient's symptoms are related to reflux episodes, although the number of these reflux episodes is not higher than normal. This situation implies that the esophagus in these subjects is hypersensitive to acid.

A limitation of a pH measurement is that reflux episodes can only be detected if these have an acidic pH. If acidic gastric secretions are mixed with food or if acid suppressant medications are used, the gastric contents can reach a neutral pH. In that situation reflux episodes are also not acidic and therefore these cannot be measured reliably with a pH sensor. However, these non-acidic reflux episodes can cause symptoms. Using impedance monitoring flow of air and fluid can be measured in the esophagus, independent of the pH of these substances. A retrograde flow of liquids suggests reflux of gastric contents, a flow in aboral direction suggests a swallow. The combination of pH and impedance monitoring thus allows detection of flow of acidic but also weakly acidic and weakly alkaline reflux. It therefore makes it possible to investigate whether the patient's

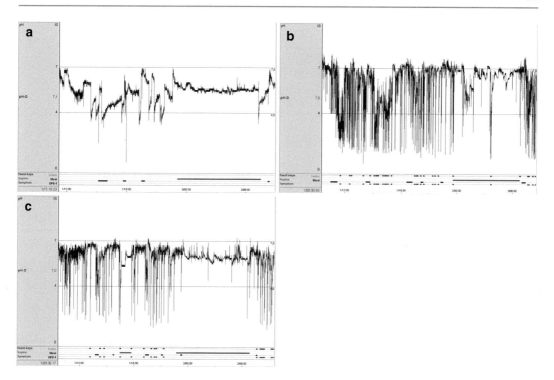

Fig. 4.14 24-hour pH measurements of the esophagus; (**a**) normal measurement, (**b**) measurement with a pathologically high esophageal acid exposure, and (**c**) measurement with normal esophageal acid exposure but during which the patient's symptoms are consistently preceded by acid reflux

symptoms are induced by weakly acidic or weakly alkaline reflux. This is particularly useful when one wants to investigate the cause of symptoms in a patient that already uses acid secretion inhibitory medication as most reflux episodes will have a pH above 4 and cannot be detected with pH monitoring alone.

4.9.4   Manometry

A low pressure of the LES and low-amplitude peristaltic contractions in the esophageal body or otherwise ineffective contractions are often seen in patients with GERD. With high-resolution manometry, often ineffective esophageal motility, fragmented peristalsis, and hiatus hernia are observed. However, these findings are not very specific for GERD. Therefore, manometry or high-resolution manometry has limited diagnostic value for GERD. However, manometry is required to determine the position of the LES and to measure the distance from the nares to the LES

in order to place a pH probe correctly, as these are placed 5 cm proximal to the upper border of the LES. Esophageal manometry is also required to exclude a severe motility disorder in patients in whom antireflux surgery is considered, as conditions such as aperistalsis are considered a contraindication for antireflux surgery. Occasionally achalasia is mistaken for GERD, because the symptoms heartburn and regurgitation may predominate. It is therefore essential to exclude achalasia by means of manometry before embarking on antireflux surgery.

4.10   Treatment of GERD

The treatment of GERD consists of several steps. The first step that is often taken by patients themselves is avoiding foods that trigger or increase symptoms such as coffee, alcohol, orange juice, peppermint, chocolate, and onions. Sometimes patients elevate the head end of the bed; this is usually advised when there are nocturnal reflux

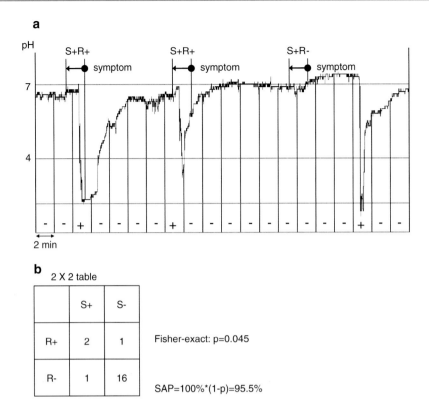

Fig. 4.15 (**a, b**) Schematic representation of the calculation of the symptom-reflux association indices. The measurement is divided into 2-min episodes; in this example 20. For each of these 2-min time windows, it is determined whether reflux occurs in it (R+) or not (R−). In this example there are 3 episodes with reflux and 17 without. The next step is counting the number of symptom events, and for each symptom it is determined whether reflux occurs prior to it or not. These numbers are entered in a two-by-two table. The number of time windows without reflux are calculated by subtracting the number of windows with reflux from the total number of 2 min windows (20 − 3 = 17). When all values are entered in the table, the Fisher Exact test is used to calculate the p-value. The symptom association probability (SAP) is 100 (p-value) times 100 %. An SAP above 95 % is considered positive, as this corresponds to a p-value of less than 0.05. The symptom index (SI) is the number of symptoms preceded by reflux divided by the total number of symptom events; in this example it is $(2/3) \times 100 \% = 66.6 \%$, which means that 66.6 % of the symptoms are reflux related

symptoms. Overweight patients benefit from losing weight, but often it is noticed that symptoms recur when their weight increases again. Smoking cessation can also be an important step in symptom control.

4.10.1 Medical Treatment of GERD

4.10.1.1   Antacids and Alginates
If lifestyle changes are insufficient, many patients will start using antacids and alginates. In almost all countries these drugs are available over the counter. Antacids neutralize gastric acid

immediately and therefore have a rapid response time. Alginates form a viscous layer on the gastric contents, which helps to reduce the number of reflux episodes. The major disadvantage of these drugs is that the effect wears off rapidly. The effect on symptoms is therefore just brief and these drugs are also not suitable for treatment of erosive reflux disease.

4.10.1.2   Histamine-2-Receptor Antagonists
Histamine-2-receptor antagonists such as ranitidine, cimetidine, and famotidine have a longer effect than antacids and alginates.

Histamine-2-receptorantagonists inhibit gastric acid secretion and result in an increase of gastric pH, which also leads to an increase in the pH of the reflux episodes. The tachyphylaxis that occurs (loss of efficacy) makes histamine-2-receptorantagonists less suitable for long-term use; their effect is partially fading after a few weeks of use. Histamine-2-receptor antagonists are effective for the treatment of reflux symptoms, but they are less effective in healing of erosive esophagitis.

4.10.1.3 Proton Pump Inhibitors

Proton pomp inhibitors (PPIs) are still considered the cornerstone of the treatment of GERD. After the introduction of omeprazole, other PPIs such as pantoprazole, rabeprazole, lansoprazole, and esomeprazole followed. PPIs inhibit gastric acid secretion more pronounced than histamine-2-receptor antagonists leading to an increase in gastric pH and reduction of the acidity of reflux episodes. During PPI treatment the total number of reflux episodes is not decreased; only the pH of the reflux episodes increases. Thus the decrease in acid reflux episodes is met by an increase in weakly acidic reflux episodes. PPIs are highly effective for the treatment of reflux symptoms, and after 8 weeks of treatment, more than 90 % of the patients with erosive esophagitis have healed. There are only few serious side effects associated with long-term PPI use. Hypomagnesemia is rarely encountered. Malabsorption is generally not clinically relevant and there is probably not an increased risk of osteoporosis and pneumonia.

After cessation of PPIs, the symptoms and esophagitis mostly recur; this is because the underlying cause of reflux disease is not taken away by the treatment. In patients with severe esophagitis and Barrett esophagus, it is therefore recommended to continue treatment lifelong; in patients with less severe abnormalities, on-demand treatment can be advised.

After intake of a PPI, the drug is rapidly absorbed in the circulation and the plasma half-life is only around 30 min. The drug can only effectively bind and block the acid-secreting cells if these are stimulated by a meal. Therefore, PPIs work optimally when taken 30 min before a meal, preferably breakfast. Newer PPIs such as dexlansoprazole have a longer plasma half-life and thus timing of intake is less critical.

4.10.2 Antireflux Surgery

GERD can be treated surgically. A fundoplication is an operation during which part of the proximal stomach is turned and fixated around the distal esophagus. This results in a cuff or wrap around the LES (Fig. 4.16). Before construction of the wrap, a hiatus hernia, if present, is corrected. If the wrap is too tight or the peristaltic reserves of the esophagus are too weak, it will result in dysphagia. There are several surgical variants of the fundoplication operation. According to the classic Nissen fundoplication, the wrap is turned 360° around the distal esophagus; with a Toupet fundoplication, a 270° wrap is created.

After a fundoplication the pressure in the LES is increased and TLESRs occur in much lower frequency, resulting in a significant decrease of reflux episodes. However, sometimes the possibility to belch is also decreased significantly which impairs venting of gastric air. Patients can complain of bloating and increased flatulence.

Indications for antireflux surgery are esophagitis and symptoms that respond insufficiently to medication. As mentioned, PPIs only reduce the acidity of reflux episodes and not reduce the number of reflux episodes. Weakly acidic reflux can also trigger heartburn and regurgitation and antireflux surgery is the only treatment that effectively reduces the number of reflux episodes. Before a patient can undergo antireflux surgery, one needs to be sure that the diagnosis of GERD is correct. An ambulatory 24-h reflux monitoring test is required, and one should be very hesitant with proceeding to surgery when there is no clear relationship between symptoms and reflux episodes during the measurement. Also, a manometry of the esophagus need to be performed to exclude major motility disorders as these can lead to severe postoperative dysphagia.

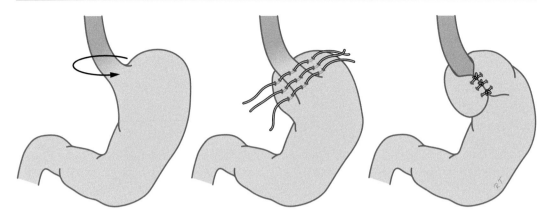

Fig. 4.16 Fundoplication according to Nissen. The proximal stomach is turned around the distal esophagus and will be stitched around the LES. A fundoplication is combined with a repair of the hiatus hernia, if present

4.11 Eosinophilic Esophagitis

Eosinophilic esophagitis (EoE) is a supposedly allergic inflammatory disorder of the esophagus, leading to progressive narrowing of the esophageal lumen. Endoscopy often shows typical changes such as esophageal narrowing, longitudinal furrows, circular rings, and edema. The disease was only first recognized in the mid 1990s. Typical symptoms of EoE are dysphagia and food impaction. There is often an overlap with GERD. EoE leads to typical endoscopic abnormalities that are clearly different from GERD (Fig. 4.17). The diagnosis of EoE is made when there are typical symptoms and a pronounced eosinophilia on esophageal biopsies in the absence of an alternative explanation.

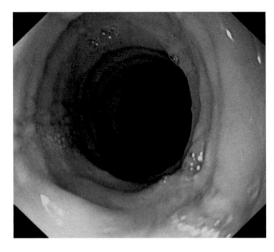

Fig. 4.17 Endoscopic image of the esophagus in a patient with eosinophilic esophagitis. Longitudinal furrows, circular rings, and edema are visible

The first step in EoE treatment is to start with a PPI in order to eliminate the role of acid reflux. The second step is immunosuppression with topical corticosteroids or dietary treatment with elimination of food for which the patient is sensitized. In case of fibrous strictures the esophagus can dilated with balloons or bougies.

4.12 Rumination Syndrome

The rumination syndrome is a behavioral disorder that is often confused with GERD. During rumination undigested food is regurgitated and this differs from vomiting as the regurgitation occurs rather effortless and is not preceded by retching. Rumination typically occurs during meals or immediately afterwards, when the regurgitated gastric contents are not acidic yet. The diagnosis of rumination syndrome used to be made based on clinical history and observations, but nowadays combined pH-impedance monitoring combined with manometry shows a typical pattern of an increase in gastric pressure immediately preceding proximally reaching reflux episodes.

4.13   **Excessive Belching**

Belching is a physiological phenomenon, but audible belching is often considered inappropriate. Excessive belching is a frequently reported symptom, often seen in combination with other disorders such as GERD and functional dyspepsia. However, belching itself can also be a reason for consultation and sometimes belching occurs as an isolated symptom. A repetitive pattern of air intake and belching is observed, sometimes more than five times per minute. The frequency of belching is often increased during stressful circumstances. Patients with excessive belching do not swallow the air but instead suck or inject the air into the esophagus using diaphragmatic or pharyngeal contractions, in the absence of swallowing with peristalsis.

Immediately after the intake of the air, it is belched out. This behavior is frequently repeated. These patients often belch audibly during the consultation. This condition used to be called aerophagia, which is Greek for air eating, but since there is no excessive swallowing of air but air suction or air injection, this term is not correct. In fact, the air will not reach the stomach, which is why it is called supragastric belching in contrast to regular gastric belching. Belching in these patients is thus not the result of regurgitation of gastric air.

It is clear that excessive belching in these patients is a behavioral disorder and the most effective treatment seems to be speech therapy or behavioral therapy, during which one tries to convince the patient that the belching is self-induced and therefore it can be learned to stop it.

5.1 Normal Gastric Function

5.1.1 Control of Gastric Motility

After its passage through the esophagus, the food bolus reaches the stomach where it is temporarily stored until grinding and further aboral transport occurs.

The functions of the proximal and the distal stomach differ considerably. The proximal part comprises the fundus and the proximal half of the gastric corpus, where smooth muscle cells have a stable membrane resting potential and where contractions are slow and tonic in nature. These properties allow the proximal stomach to serve as a reservoir for the meal. In the distal part of the stomach, which comprises the antrum and the distal half of the corpus, smooth muscle cells display spontaneous oscillations of the membrane potential at a frequency of 3 cycles/min (the so-called slow waves). Slow waves are generated in the corpus near the greater curvature, in the pacemaker region of the stomach. Slow waves arise in the interstitial cells of Cajal, and they determine the rhythm at which phasic contractions in the distal stomach can occur (Fig. 5.1). Slow waves are continuously present, even when the distal stomach is not contracting. Contractions occur during the most depolarized phase of the slow waves and are triggered by the release of excitatory neurotransmitters from myenteric nerve endings.

In the stomach, similar to the rest of the gastrointestinal tract, the myenteric plexus is located between the circular and the longitudinal muscle layer. Although myenteric neurons receive input from the central nervous system through parasympathetic (vagus nerve) and sympathetic autonomic nerves, the enteric nervous system is able to function independently. The vagus nerve plays mainly an afferent or sensory role, as 80–90 % of vagal nerves convey information from the gastrointestinal tract to the brain.

Afferent information from the gastrointestinal tract is integrated in the brain stem (especially the tractus solitarius) and influences myenteric plexus activity through efferent pathways. These so-called vago-vagal reflexes play a major role in the control of gastric motility, both during the fed and the fasting state. The sympathetic innervation mainly inhibits the release of acetylcholine from the myenteric plexus.

Gastric function is also controlled by a variety of gastrointestinal hormones. They mainly originate from the small intestine, where the release of many different gut peptides is controlled by the presence or absence of nutrients. These hormones signal to the brain for the control of hunger and satiety, while at the same time adapting gastric function to the presence or anticipated presence of food.

© Springer International Publishing Switzerland 2016
A.J. Bredenoord et al., *A Guide to Gastrointestinal Motility Disorders*,
DOI 10.1007/978-3-319-26938-2_5

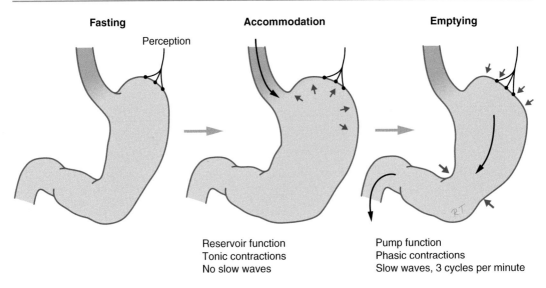

Fasting	Accommodation	Emptying

Perception

Reservoir function   Pump function
Tonic contractions   Phasic contractions
No slow waves   Slow waves, 3 cycles per minute

Fig. 5.1 Gastric motility during fasting, during food ingestion (accommodation), and during gastric emptying (Published with kind permission of © Rogier Trompert Medical Art 2015)

5.1.2   Fasting or Interdigestive Motility

During fasting, the stomach and small intestine exhibit a recurrent pattern of contractions and quiescence, which is called the migrating motor complex (MMC). A cycle of the MMC lasts 90–120 min and consists of 3 distinct phases (see also Chaps. 1 and 6). Phase I is a period of absent contractile activity; during phase II contractions occur at highly variable frequency and without coordination. Phase III is characterized by a period of approximately 5 min of maximal contractile frequency (3/min in the stomach), which is again followed by phase I. This contraction pattern starts proximally, in the stomach or duodenum, and migrates distally over the small intestine to start again proximally. During the passage of phase III in the gastric antrum, nondigested particles are cleared from the stomach. Phase III in the gastric antrum is also associated with an intense hunger sensation and may play a role in the control of food intake.

5.1.3   Postprandial Motility

The MMC is interrupted by food intake. Driven by the extrinsic innervation, the gastrointestinal

tract switches to the so-called postprandial motility pattern. In the stomach, this is characterized by relaxation of the proximal stomach and coordinated contractions in the distal stomach (Fig. 5.1).

Following each deglutition, the lower esophageal sphincter and the proximal stomach relax to facilitate passage and arrival of the food bolus in the gastric corpus. The deglutitive relaxation of the proximal stomach, which is associated with inhibition of antral contractile activity, is called *receptive relaxation.* Gastric filling with a meal is not associated with a rise in intragastric pressure owing to a second type of relaxation of the proximal stomach, which is called *adaptive relaxation.* Both types of relaxation generate *gastric accommodation, which represents the food reservoir function of the stomach,* which is largely coordinated through a vago-vagal reflex pathway. As the meal becomes increasingly fragmented by gastric grinding (see below), a rise in tone of the proximal stomach occurs, which will help to promote the process of gastric emptying.

Shortly after ingestion of the meal, peristaltic contractions occur in the distal stomach, propagating from mid-corpus to the pylorus. Upon arrival of this contraction wave at the pylorus, the latter closes briefly, resulting in the food bolus being thrown back to a more proximal part of the stomach. This process helps to grind the food to small particles. As soon as these fragments are small enough, passage through the pylorus to the duodenum occurs. Hence, the pylorus functions as a filter for larger particles and thus plays a key role in the control of gastric emptying.

5.1.4 Control of Gastric Emptying

A large number of physiological mechanisms are involved in the control of gastric emptying, resulting in a different handling of liquids and solids. Liquids empty with an exponential curve, with increasing caloric and osmotic density slowing down empting. It is the pressure gradient between the stomach and the duodenum which drives the liquid emptying rate, with tone of the proximal stomach and resistance at the pylorus as the most important variables (Fig. 5.2).

Emptying of solids follows a different pattern. In an initial phase, the antral peristaltic pump grinds the food, and no emptying occurs. This phase is called the "lag phase." As soon as particles of 1 mm diameter or less are generated, passage through the pylorus occurs, and the emptying follows an almost linear curve (Fig. 5.3).

Pyloric passage of food occurs in a pulsatile fashion and is controlled by hormonal and neural feedback from the duodenum. Small intestinal receptors sensitive to pH, osmolarity, fatty acid chain length and concentrations of glucose, and L-tryptophan will slow gastric emptying through neural (enteric nerves) or hormonal (glucagon-like peptide 1 (Figs. 5.4 and 5.5), cholecystokinin, peptide YY, and others) signaling. In addition, there is also some colonic negative feedback, as colonic filling slows down gastric emptying.

5.2 Gastric Motility Disorders

5.2.1 Symptoms

Symptoms that are associated with disorders of gastric motility are not specific and include postprandial fullness, early satiation, upper abdominal bloating, nausea, vomiting, anorexia, and epigastric pain. In severe cases this may lead to weight loss and inability for sufficient nutrition through the oral route. These symptoms may also occur in a large number of disorders of the upper gastrointestinal tract or even the pancreatico-hepatobiliary system. Furthermore, the relationship between symptom pattern, symptom severity, and underlying gastric motility disorders is often poor. It is also assumed that disordered gastric emptying contributes to poor glycemic control in patients with diabetes mellitus.

5.2.2 Gastroparesis

5.2.2.1 Definition and Causes
Gastroparesis is defined by the presence of severely delayed emptying in the absence of mechanical obstruction. Hence, in a first phase, a mechanical factor needs to be excluded by means of gastroduodenoscopy or radiological examina-

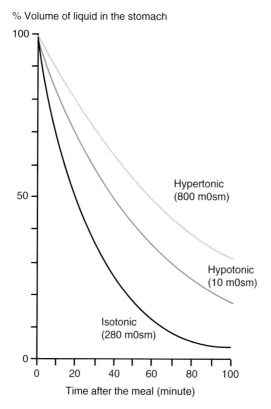

Fig. 5.2 The effect of the osmotic density of a liquid meal on the rate of gastric emptying

Fig. 5.3 Radioisotope gastric emptying scintigraphy, with quantification of the amount of tracer present in the stomach region over time

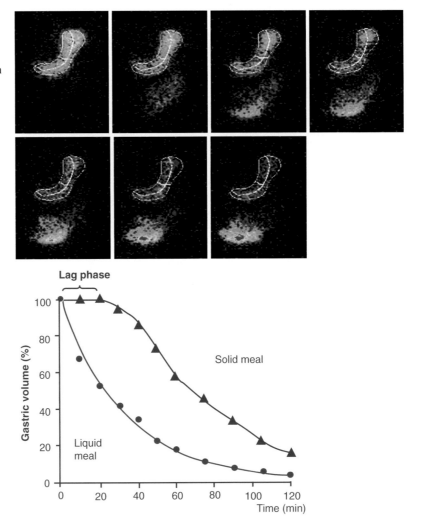

tion (small bowel X-ray, CT, or MR enterography). Gastroparesis can occur as a consequence of multiple and diverse conditions. A number of drugs can induce or worsen gastroparesis, especially anticholinergics, opioids, L-dopa, tricyclic antidepressants, and phenothiazines. In these cases, if possible, this type of medication should be interrupted. Besides medication, the most important causes of gastroparesis are diabetes mellitus and postsurgical gastroparesis. More rarely, a number of metabolic or neurological conditions, anorexia nervosa, connective tissue disorders, and chronic intestinal pseudo-obstruction may also be associated with gastroparesis. However, in the largest group of gastroparesis patients, no underlying cause is

identified and these are referred to as having idiopathic gastroparesis.

Gastroparesis occurs in both type 1 and type 2 diabetes, but the highest prevalence is found in type 1 diabetes patients with autonomic neuropathy and poor glycemic control. Hyperglycemia alone is already able to slow down gastric emptying and, conversely, delayed gastric emptying may impair optimal glycemic control in insulin-treated diabetes. In the large group of idiopathic gastroparesis patients, a subset has a history suggestive of triggering by a viral infection. Surgery, especially when affecting vagal integrity, impairs control of gastric motility resulting in rapid emptying of liquids (which may lead to dumping syndrome, see below) and delayed emptying of solids. Gastric

%Volume of liquid in the stomach

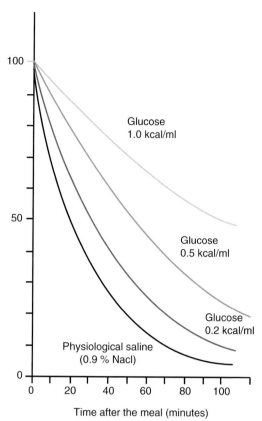

Fig. 5.4 The effect of the caloric content of a liquid meal on the rate of gastric emptying

% Volume of nutrient in the stomach

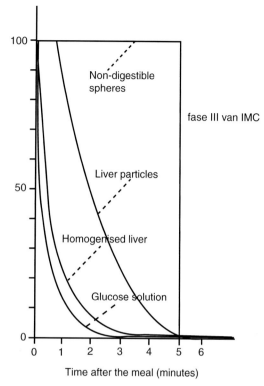

Fig. 5.5 The effect of the particle size of a meal on the rate of gastric emptying. Large particles needed to be reduced in size before they can pass the pylorus. Nondigestible particles are the last ones to exit the stomach

emptying rate is also significantly delayed in patients with anorexia nervosa, possibly as a consequence of malnutrition and muscular atrophy.

5.2.2.2 Diagnosis

In patients presenting with symptoms suggestive of gastroparesis, mechanical, endocrine (e.g., thyroid dysfunction, adrenal insufficiency), or electrolyte disorders need to be excluded. Drugs that could induce delayed gastric emptying should be stopped if possible (Tables 5.1 and 5.2).

A number of methodologies are available for the measurement of gastric emptying rate. In clinical practice, mainly radio-scintigraphy and stable isotope breath tests are used. Antral hypomotility can also be documented by manometry, but this is rarely applied clinically.

The scintigraphic gastric emptying test is internationally still considered the gold standard test, but this is influenced by the fact that gastric emptying breath test only recently received approval in the United States. For the scintigraphic emptying test, the subject ingests a meal which contains the radioisotope label, whose presence in the stomach can be detected by the gamma camera. Gastric emptying is measured as the decline in radioactive counts in the stomach area over time (Fig. 5.2). Accuracy of the test requires measurement up to 4 h after meal ingestion.

Both a solid and a liquid meal can be labeled, or both can be combined using different tracers. The methods are limited by the use of radioactive labels, a relatively high cost, and a poor standardization of the test meal across centers.

Table 5.1 Causes of delayed gastric emptying

Acute
Peritonitis, acute abdominal pain, inflammation
Postoperative state
Gastritis, infections, gastroenteritis
Metabolic disorders: hyperglycemia, acidosis, hyper- and hypocalcemia
Chronic
Idiopathic
Nerve damage caused by:
Diabetes
Malignant infiltration
Vagotomy
Infection (*Trypanosoma cruzi*)
Smooth muscle disorders (scleroderma, polymyositis, amyloidosis, etc.)
Neurologic disorders (stroke, Parkinson, multiple sclerosis)
Hypothyroidism
Anorexia nervosa
Chronic intestinal pseudo-obstruction
Psychogenic vomiting
Acute and chronic
Mechanical obstruction
Drug induced (opioids, anticholinergics, antihypertensives, tricyclic antidepressants, levodopa, GLP-1 analogues, amylin)
Pregnancy
Tabes dorsalis

Table 5.2 Causes of rapid gastric emptying

Vagotomy
Partial gastrectomy
Hyperthyroidism
Exocrine pancreatic insufficiency
Zollinger-Ellison syndrome

An alternative approach is the measurement of gastric emptying based on exhaled $^{13}CO_2$. For this test, a meal is ingested which contains a ^{13}C-labeled substance, such as octanoic acid, acetic acid, or *Spirulina platensis*. When this substance enters the duodenum, it is rapidly absorbed, and after hepatic metabolization, $^{13}CO_2$ is exhaled. By taking breath samples at regular intervals after ingestion of the meal, mathematical processing of the $^{13}CO_2$ content generates a curve which allows to quantify gastric emptying rate. The ^{13}C isotope is nonradioactive, and the test meal and measurement can be taken at a table. Also for this test, there is a lack of standardization of the meal. Probably also here a 4-h measurement is optimal.

5.2.2.3 Treatment

Once a diagnosis of gastroparesis has been made, the most frequent approach is to start treatment with a gastroprokinetic agent. If nausea is a prominent symptom, metoclopramide or domperidone can be used. However, metoclopramide has been associated with neurological side effects (pseudoparkinsonism), and domperidone has been associated with QT interval prolongation. For these reasons, only standard doses should be used, and domperidone should not be combined with other drugs that prolong QT interval and avoided in patients with a (family) history of cardiac arrhythmias. Until 2002, cisapride was often used in this indication, but this drug was withdrawn because of arrhythmias related to QT prolongation. Erythromycin, at low doses, is a potent gastroprokinetic agent through its motilin receptor agonist properties. Long-term efficacy in generating symptomatic benefit is less certain for erythromycin, and also this drug can prolong the QT interval. Mechanistic and pilot data suggest potential efficacy of prucalopride in gastroparesis, but more studies are needed. A number of novel agents, including agonists at the ghrelin and motilin receptor, are under evaluation for the treatment of gastroparesis.

In case of failure of medical therapy and relevant weight loss, intestinal tube feeding can be considered. Food is administered via a nasointestinal tube or via a percutaneous jejunostomy tube, thereby bypassing the stomach. The use of a gastric electrical stimulator (based on an implantable neurostimulator) is popular for the treatment of severe gastroparesis in the United States. However, controlled trials failed to provide convincing evidence of efficacy. In exceptional cases, partial or total gastrectomy has been reported as a treatment approach for refractory debilitating gastroparesis, but results are unpredictable and there is a major risk of postoperative dumping syndrome (see below).

5.2.3 Functional Dyspepsia

5.2.3.1 Definition and Diagnosis

Functional dyspepsia is defined as the presence of symptoms thought to originate from the gastro-duodenal region, in the absence of an underlying organic abnormality that explains the symptoms. Dyspeptic symptoms in the broad sense comprise early satiation, postprandial fullness, and pain or burning in the stomach region and may also be accompanied by upper abdominal bloating, nausea, or belching. An upper gastrointestinal endoscopy is the key examination in patients presenting with such symptoms in whom further diagnostic exploration is warranted. In the vast majority of these patients (70 %), no endoscopic abnormalities are found, and in the absence of bothersome typical reflux symptoms, a diagnosis of "functional dyspepsia" can be made. In clinical practice, routine blood laboratory tests are also performed, but the diagnostic yield in patients without alarm symptoms (weight loss, nocturnal pain, blood loss in the stools, anemia) is low. In high-prevalence areas, celiac disease can be excluded by measuring transglutaminase antibodies or a related test. An abdominal ultrasound is also often performed in patients with dyspeptic symptoms, but large case series show that this is only cost-effective in case of colicky upper abdominal pain, to rule out gallstone disease.

5.2.3.2 Pathophysiological Concepts

In spite of its high prevalence, the pathogenesis of functional dyspepsia remains unknown. Most likely, this is a multifactorial condition which arises in patients with a genetic predisposition and can be triggered by acute gastrointestinal infections and modulated by psychosocial and immunological factors. No diagnostic test for functional dyspepsia exists. Accompanying disorders of gastric sensorimotor function can be demonstrated in subsets of functional dyspepsia patients, including delayed gastric emptying rate with antral hypomotility, impaired gastric accommodation (proximal storage function during and after meal intake), or hypersensitivity to gastric distention. In the duodenum, signs of low-grade inflammation can be found, such as increased numbers of eosinophils and mast cells and lymphoid cell aggregates, and this is especially the case in patients whose functional dyspepsia started after an acute gastroenteritis. However, the correlation between all of these function disorders and symptom pattern or severity is poor.

An area of controversy is the role of *Helicobacter pylori* in the pathogenesis of dyspeptic symptoms. The presence of *Helicobacter* infection can be detected by measuring antibodies in blood, by demonstrating presence of the antigen in feces, by direct demonstration of the presence of *Helicobacter* in biopsies obtained at endoscopy, or with the urease breath test. While the causal role of *Helicobacter* in peptic ulcer disease is well established, its role in generating dyspeptic symptoms with negative endoscopy is less clear. The presence of helicobacter does not lead to significant alterations in gastric motility or sensitivity, and eradication of helicobacter does not improve dyspeptic symptoms in the short term. Nevertheless, a small subset (1 in 15) of helicobacter-infected patients with dyspeptic symptoms and negative endoscopy becomes asymptomatic during longer (1 year) follow-up after eradication, indicating a potential but limited pathogenetic role for the infection.

Equally controversial is the role of psychosocial factors in functional dyspepsia patients. It is clear that psychological factors can alter gastric function through efferent autonomic nerves and through activation of the hypothalamo-pituitary-adrenal axis. Hence, it is highly likely that psychological factors such as anxiety, depression, somatization, and stress play a role in the severity and fluctuations of functional dyspepsia symptoms. The extent to which this aspect should drive therapy remains to be established.

5.2.3.3 Treatment

Not all functional dyspepsia patients require pharmacotherapy. Reassuring explanation and normal findings at, for instance, endoscopy can eliminate any worries about underlying potentially serious medical conditions. Often, a number of lifestyle adjustments such as regular smaller meals with low lipid content, exercise, and avoidance of caffeine and other stimulants are recommended, but their therapeutic impact has not been proven.

Proton pump inhibitors are often the first-line pharmacotherapeutic approach to functional dyspepsia, especially when epigastric pain or burning is the predominant symptom or when the patient also experiences heartburn. In case of postprandial fullness or early satiation as predominant symptom, the chance of favorable response to acid-suppressive therapy is considerably decreased. In this case prokinetic agents can be used. However, there is a paucity of prokinetic agents with proven efficacy and safety and worldwide availability. In Europe, South America, and the Far East, specific prokinetics, usually dopamine-2 receptor antagonists such as domperidone or 5-HT$_4$ receptor agonists such as clebopride or mosapride, are often available. Tricyclic antidepressants can be used in refractory cases, but they will also be most beneficial in case of predominant epigastric pain or burning or perhaps in case of major psychosocial comorbidity. Selective noradrenaline/serotonin reuptake inhibitors are not very useful in treating functional dyspepsia symptoms and are not well tolerated. There is also evidence that some herbal preparations, such as Iberogast® in Europe and Rikkunshito in Japan, are effective in functional dyspepsia.

5.2.4 Dumping Syndrome

5.2.4.1 Definition

Dumping syndrome is a constellation of symptoms and reactions that occur when the small intestine is exposed to excessive amounts of nutrients (Fig. 5.6). It is a frequently occurring complication of total or partial gastrectomy or of vagotomy as performed in the past as a treatment for peptic ulcer disease. Dumping syndrome also occurs in up to 50 % of patients who underwent subtotal or distal esophagectomy, probably because of loss of control of gastric emptying by the vagus nerve. Dumping syndrome can also occur as a complication of antireflux fundoplication. In recent years, dumping mainly occurs as a consequence of partial gastrectomy in bariatric surgery.

Symptoms of dumping syndrome can be divided in early dumping symptoms, where cardiovascular

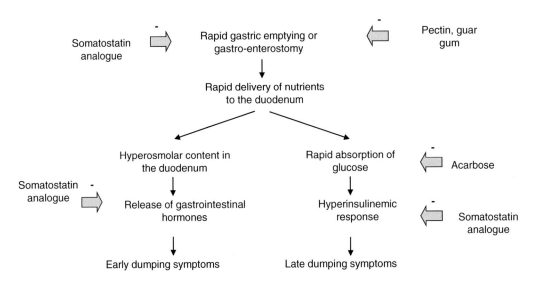

Fig. 5.6 Pathophysiology and therapeutic targets in dumping syndrome

(palpitations, tachycardia, transpiration, flushing, pre-syncope) and abdominal symptoms (abdominal pain, diarrhea, nausea, cramps) occur, and a late dumping phase which is identical to hypoglycemia (hunger, weakness, transpiration, tremor, loss of concentration up to syncope).

5.2.4.2 Diagnosis

The diagnosis is based on typical symptoms in a patient with a history of upper gastrointestinal surgery. Usually endoscopy and radiographies are performed to rule out stenosis or other mechanical factors after surgery. Diagnostic certainty can be obtained by a glucose tolerance test, where at each glycemia sampling point also pulse rate and hematocrit are determined. A diagnosis of dumping syndrome is confirmed in case of an early rise in hematocrit (10 % of original value) or pulse rate (>10 beats per minute) or a late hypoglycemia (<60 mg/dl). This diagnostic test is specific but not very sensitive. In case of late dumping, measurement of hypoglycemia during symptoms can also confirm the diagnosis.

5.2.4.3 Treatment

The first step in treating dumping syndrome is a diet poor in rapidly absorbable carbohydrates, with smaller more frequent meals and avoidance of drinking during meals. If this is not sufficient, acarbose, an inhibitor of generation and uptake of monosaccharides, can be taken with meals. In case of important early dumping symptoms, increasing the viscosity of the meal by adding guar gum or pectin can be tried, but patient compliance is often poor because of the unpleasant taste of these agents. In refractory cases, short-acting somatostatin analogues can be injected subcutaneously prior to each meal, or a slow-release preparation can be injected every 4 weeks. Complications of somatostatin analogue therapy are gallbladder stone formation and steatorrhea.

Small Bowel

6

6.1 Small Bowel Motility

During fasting, the stomach and small bowel exhibit a recurrent pattern of contractions and quiescence, which is called the migrating motor complex (MMC). A full MMC cycle lasts 90–120 min and comprises three phases (see Chap. 1). Phase 1 is a period of absence of contractions; during phase II contractions occur with highly variable frequency without apparent rigorous organization. Phase III is characterized by a period of 5–12 min of strong contractions at maximum frequency (3/min in the stomach, up to 12/min in the small intestine), followed again by phase I. This pattern starts proximally, in the stomach or the duodenum, and gradually moves aborally to the distal small bowel, to start again proximally. During the passage of phase III, non-absorbable remnants are cleared from the antrum, and intestinal phase III ensures further evacuation of small bowel content into the large intestine. This activity is referred to as the intestinal housekeeper function of the MMC.

Upon food ingestion, small bowel motility switches to a so-called postprandial motor pattern. In this phase, apparently random contractile activity occurs throughout the small intestine. However, the composition of the meal and its fiber content and viscosity have all been shown to influence the type of contractions. The control of postprandial motility is very poorly understood and understudied.

6.2 Disorders of Small Bowel Motility

The small bowel is the largest segment of the gastrointestinal tract but is less frequently studied. Disorders of small bowel motility are part of a spectrum (Fig. 6.1). In frequently occurring conditions, such as functional dyspepsia or the irritable bowel syndrome, subtle abnormalities in small bowel motility, with uncertain pathophysiological significance, can be observed. Severe disorders, such as chronic intestinal pseudo-obstruction, are rare (Table 6.1).

6.2.1 Frequently Occurring Disorders of Small Bowel Motility of Uncertain Pathophysiological Significance

In a large group of gastrointestinal disorders, changes in small bowel motility are present, but it is unclear to which extent they contribute to symptom generation. The abnormalities mainly refer to changes in frequency and propagation of phase III of the migrating motor complex. Such relatively subtle changes in small bowel motility have been reported in the irritable bowel syndrome and in functional dyspepsia, but these conditions are addressed in detail in Chaps. 5 and 7.

© Springer International Publishing Switzerland 2016
A.J. Bredenoord et al., *A Guide to Gastrointestinal Motility Disorders*,
DOI 10.1007/978-3-319-26938-2_6

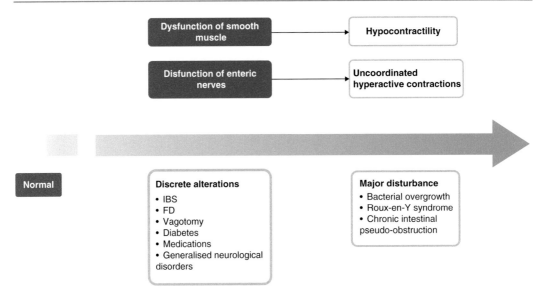

Fig. 6.1 Spectrum of disorders of small bowel motility

Table 6.1 Motility disorders of the small intestine

Acute
Infectious gastroenteritis
Paralytic ileus as a complication of:
Ketoacidosis
Hypokalemia
Peritonitis
Postoperative state
Chronic
Functional dyspepsia
Irritable bowel syndrome
Hyperthyroidism
Pseudo-obstruction:
As part of chronic idiopathic intestinal pseudo-obstruction (CIIP)
Secondary to diabetes, scleroderma

Small bowel motility is also altered after surgery of the upper gastrointestinal tract. After vagotomy, as a consequence of partial or total gastrectomy or esophagectomy, conversion of interdigestive motility to the fed state upon meal ingestion may be lost. Rarely, after Roux-en-Y construction, retrograde peristalsis may occur in the efferent loop when a distal pacemaker is dominant over more proximally located pacemakers. This entity can only be diagnosed by manometry.

Finally, in diabetic neuropathy or after large vascular graft surgery in the abdomen, probably because of a loss of inhibitory innervation, hypermotility and suppression of phase I of the migrating motor complex can be observed.

6.2.2 Chronic Intestinal Pseudo-obstruction

Chronic intestinal pseudo-obstruction comprises a group of rare, severe disorders of gastrointestinal motility. The diagnosis is made when a clinical picture suggestive of obstruction (dilated small bowel, air-fluid levels) occurs in the absence of a mechanical cause, based on endoscopic, radiological, and sometimes surgical evaluation (Fig. 6.2).

These disorders are caused by severe disorders of smooth muscle function or of the intrinsic innervation or of interstitial cells of Cajal in the small intestine. Both sporadic and hereditary types of chronic intestinal pseudo-obstruction exist, and the disorder can be primary but also secondary, as part of a generalized muscular (e.g., mitochondrial myopathy) or neural (e.g., amyloidosis) disease.

With the exception of generalized disorders as mentioned above, making a diagnosis will some-

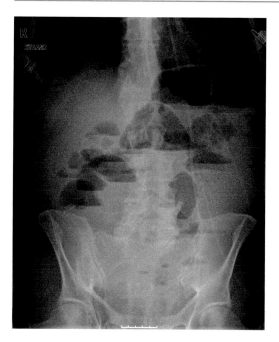

Fig. 6.2 Abdominal X-ray of a patient with chronic idiopathic intestinal pseudo-obstruction. Numerous air-fluid levels are present in the small intestine, as well as a single dilated small bowel loop. A plain abdominal X-ray examination does not allow to distinguish idiopathic pseudo-obstruction from mechanic ileus

times even require obtaining a transmural small bowel biopsy, which allows morphologic evaluation of neuromuscular structures. This can reveal degenerative or inflammatory neuromuscular disorders. One condition worth mentioning is idiopathic myenteric ganglionitis, which is characterized by an inflammatory infiltrate around the myenteric plexus and increased neuronal apoptosis, which may respond to immunosuppressive therapy. These patients often have circulating anti-Hu antibodies, which may be screened for as a routine test.

Small bowel manometry can be suggestive of major neural or muscular dysfunction in case of (suspected) pseudo-obstruction (Fig. 6.3). In typical myopathy cases, contractions of low amplitude occur but the contractile pattern is usually preserved, if still evaluable. In case of neuropathies, contractions of normal amplitude occur, but their control and organization are lacking. This can be apparent as a loss of shift to fed motility pattern after a meal, disordered organization, propagation, or coordination of the MMC, including long-lasting hypercontractility in individual segments

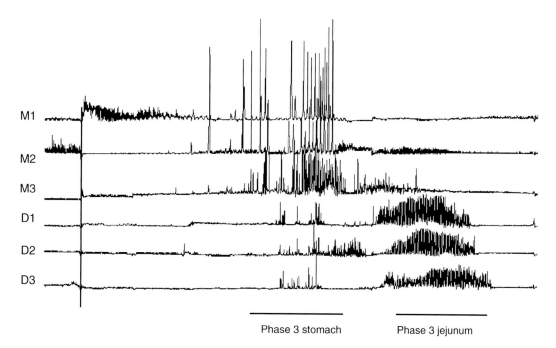

Phase 3 stomach   Phase 3 jejunum

Fig. 6.3 Interdigestive motility, measured with 3 sensors in the stomach (*M1-3*) and 3 in the small bowel (*D1-3*). The segment displays phase 3 contractions that start from the stomach and migrate to the small intestine. They are followed by phase 1 (quiescence). *MMC* migrating motor complex (so-called bursts). In disorders of interstitial cells of Cajal, a myopathy-like picture can occur.

Due to the rarity of this condition, treatment of intestinal pseudo-obstruction is difficult and mainly based on experience and clinical tradition, rather than on controlled studies. Therapy usually involves administration of drugs that enhance gastrointestinal motility, antibiotics to treat bacterial overgrowth if present (see below), and agents that limit gastrointestinal secretions (acid-suppressive therapy, somatostatin analogues). In extreme cases, partial resection or small intestinal derivation stomas may be necessary, and some patients depend on liquid nutrients or chronic parenteral nutrition to maintain body weight.

6.2.3 Small Intestinal Bacterial Overgrowth

While the colon contains high numbers of commensal bacteria, their number is substantially less in the small intestine. This is at least in part attributable to the effect of phase 3 of the MMC, as absence of phase 3 predisposes to small intestinal bacterial overgrowth. Small intestinal bacterial overgrowth is facilitated by chronic PPI use and occurs readily in intestinal segments that are excluded from normal transit (so-called blind loop syndrome), for instance, after a Roux-en-Y anastomosis.

The gold standard for diagnosing small intestinal bacterial overgrowth is aspiration and culture from the lumen, but this is somewhat invasive and technically difficult. In clinical practice, the diagnosis is usually made using breath tests. The principle relies on measurement of the speed with which degradation products of ingested substances that are metabolized by bacteria appear in the breath. Substrates that can be used include glucose, lactulose, or bile acids, and these can be labeled with a stable isotope that is measured in the breath, or the H2 content in the breath is measured after administration of unlabeled glucose or lactulose.

Treatment of bacterial overgrowth consists of intermittent short antibiotic courses, with alternating choices of antibiotics. Prokinetic agents can be used additionally.

6.2.4 Mechanical Sub-occlusion and Intestinal Motility

The diagnosis of mechanical factors that obstruct small intestinal transit relies on endoscopy (for the gastroduodenal segment) and especially on radiology (small bowel X-ray or CT or MR enteroclysis) (Fig. 6.4). In rare cases, imaging may fail to demonstrate a substenosing lesion, and in these cases small bowel manometry may show a pattern that is highly suggestive of mechanical subobstruction. In such cases, a typical pattern of simultaneous repetitive contractions occurs over a long segment of small bowel, separated by brief quiescence episodes. This so-called pattern of "minute rhythm" or "clustered contractions" shows the attempt of the small

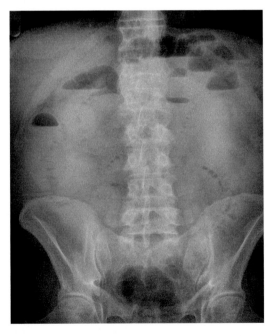

Fig. 6.4 Abdominal X-ray of patient with ileus. Multiple small intestinal air-fluid levels can be seen

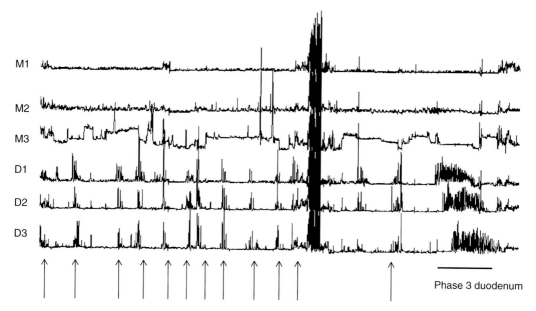

M1

M2

M3

D1

D2

D3

Phase 3 duodenum

Fig. 6.5 Gastroduodenal manometry pattern suggestive of mechanical obstruction. Gastric contractions (*M1-3*) are normal, but "clustered contractions" (*arrows*) occur in the duodenum (*D1-3*). A duodenal phase 3 occurs toward the end of the tracing. The cause was attributed to a partial malrotation with compressive effect on the distal duodenum

intestine to overcome the obstructing segment through strong peristaltic activity (Fig. 6.5). When this pattern is present during the vast majority of the measurement period, this is strongly suggestive of mechanical obstruction which may lead to additional radiological imaging or surgical exploration.

Colon

7

7.1 Introduction

The most important function of the colon is to reabsorb water and electrolytes from the liquid chyme that arrives from the small bowel. Under normal circumstances approximately 1500 ml of chyme is delivered to the cecum per day. After reabsorption only 150 ml remains (Fig. 7.1).

In addition to the reabsorption function, the colon also has an important storage function. The feces that is produced during the course of one or several days can remain stored in the colon until a suitable moment for defecation occurs.

For the execution of the abovementioned tasks, the colon not only needs a sufficiently large absorbing surface, but also movements of the wall of the organ. Moreover, specialized functions of the pelvic floor, the anal sphincters, and the rectum are required, but these will be discussed in Chap. 8 of this book.

7.2 Anatomy and Innervation

The human colon is 1–1.5 m long. The organ usually has more curves and bends than are depicted in the anatomy books. From proximal to distal, the cecum, the ascending colon, the transverse colon, the sigmoid, and the rectum are distinguished (Fig. 7.2).

Like the other parts of the digestive canal, the colon has an outer longitudinal and an inner cir-cular muscle layer. However, in the colon the longitudinal layer is not equally distributed over the circumference. Most longitudinal muscle fibers are found in three longitudinal bands known as taeniae (singular: taenia). Along the length of the colon, with the exception of the rectum, the colon has circular indentations with saccular pouches in between. These are called haustra (singular: haustrum). As in the other parts of the canal the wall of the colon contains neuronal plexuses, such as the myenteric and the submucosal plexus. The parasympathetic fibers that reach the right part of the colon are branches of the vagus nerve. The left part of the colon receives its parasympathetic innervation via the pelvic splanchnic nerves. The orthosympathetic innervation of the colon is supplied via perivascular plexuses.

The motility of the colon is regulated not only neurally but also hormonally. The most important hormones that stimulate colonic motility are gastrin and cholecystokinin. The most important inhibitory hormones are glucagon and vasoactive intestinal polypeptide (VIP).

7.3 Colonic Motility

Two types of colonic contractile patterns can be distinguished. These are haustrating (segmenting) contractions and mass contractions, also known as "high-amplitude propagated contractions" (HAPCs) (Fig. 7.3).

© Springer International Publishing Switzerland 2016
A.J. Bredenoord et al., *A Guide to Gastrointestinal Motility Disorders*,
DOI 10.1007/978-3-319-26938-2_7

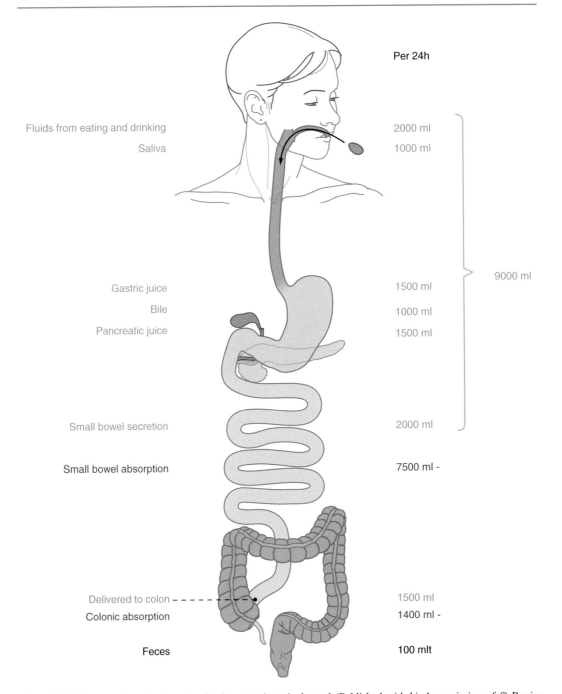

Fig. 7.1 Fluid secretion and absorption in the gastrointestinal canal (Published with kind permission of © Rogier Trompert Medical Art 2015)

Fig. 7.3 Schematic representation of the two types of colonic contractions (Published with kind permission of © Rogier Trompert Medical Art 2015)

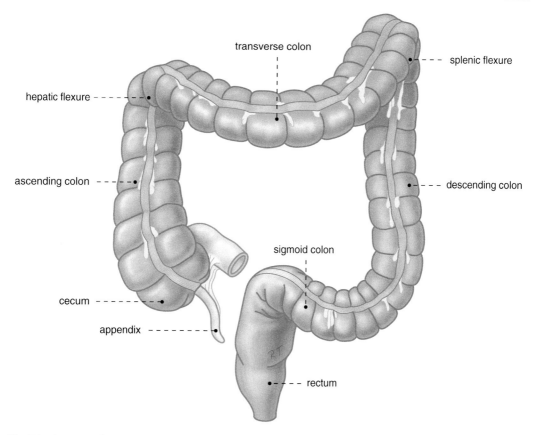

Fig. 7.2   Anatomy of the colon (Published with kind permission of © Rogier Trompert Medical Art 2015)

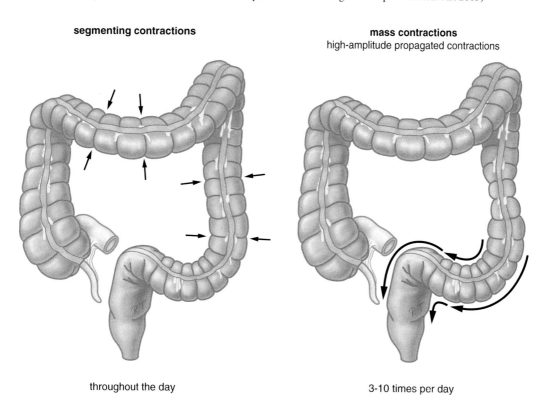

7.3.1 Haustrating Contractions

The haustrating contractions are brought about by local contractions of the circular muscle layer. Many of the haustrating contractions are stationary or almost stationary. They give the colon its typical haustrated appearance. The movements of these contractions are so slow that during short observations one gets the impression that the haustrated appearance of the colon is based on preformed anatomical structures. Prolonged observations of colonic appearance on X-ray have made clear however that the characteristic haustration pattern changes continuously.

Using intraluminal manometry the haustrating contractions can be recognized as pressure waves of variable duration and amplitude, without a clearly recognizable rhythm (Fig. 7.4). Electromyographic studies of the colon have shown that electrical slow waves are present, but, unlike the situation in the small bowel, these lack regularity. Often multiple slow wave frequencies coexist in the colon.

The haustrating contractions of the colon do not lead to significant displacements of colonic contents. Their primary function is to mix and triturate the contents, enabling optimal contact with the mucosa. This ensures that the resorption of water and salts is optimal. The frequency and amplitude of haustrating contractions increase after a meal, and haustrating contractions almost cease during the night.

7.3.2 Mass Contractions

Mass contractions are powerful, prolonged circular contractions that travel in the direction of the anus. When studied manometrically, the pressure in the lumen of the colon is found to reach values of several hundreds of mmHg during these contractions. Hence, the alternative name high-

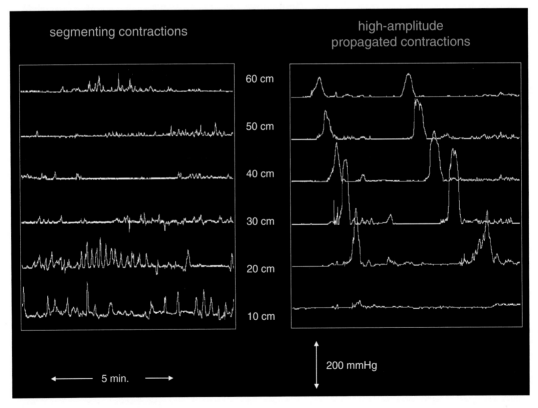

Fig. 7.4 Manometric recordings of the two types of colonic contractions. *Left* segmenting contractions, *right* high-amplitude peristaltic contractions

amplitude peristaltic contractions (HAPCs). The propagation speed of the contractions is about 1 cm per second. HAPCs do not occur frequently; in the human colon about 6 HAPCs contractions can be seen per day. They occur preferentially in the morning after awakening, after breakfast, and after meals. HAPCs effectively propel colonic contents in the direction of the anus. When feces arrives in the rectum, a sensation of urgency can arise and defecation may follow.

7.4   Postprandial versus Interdigestive Activity

The interdigestive migrating motor complex (MMC) that is the hallmark of fasting state motility in the stomach and small intestine is absent in the colon. Nevertheless, there are differences between interdigestive and postprandial motor activities in the colon. Within minutes after ingestion of a meal the motility of the colon increases significantly. This so-called gastrocolonic response lasts 30–60 min. During the gastrocolonic response the incidence and amplitude of the haustrating contractions is increased. In addition, the meal may elicit one or more mass contractions. The gastrocolonic response is mediated by release of the hormones cholecystokinin and gastrin, but an increased activation via the autonomic nervous system also plays a role.

7.5   Symptoms of Disordered Colonic Motility and Perception

Disordered motility of the colon can lead to constipation, diarrhea, and abdominal pain. When colonic visceral sensitivity is increased, pain is the predominant symptom, but the feeling of a distended abdomen (bloating) may also arise.

7.5.1   Constipation

It is difficult to define constipation. In fact, constipation comprises a variable assortment of symptoms. In the past often a low defecation frequency (fewer than three defecations per week) was used to define constipation. We now accept that constipation can also be present when defecation frequency is in the normal range. It has also been proposed to use fecal weight (in grams per 24 h) as an objective criterion for constipation. A production of less than 100 g would be abnormal. However, this criterion is difficult to use in daily practice. Many patients with constipation do not complain of a low frequency of defecation, and hardly any patient would report a low fecal weight. Rather, the patients' presenting symptoms are hard stools, the feeling of incomplete evacuation, or the necessity to use straining (Table 7.1). In the Rome III classification all of these symptoms are taken into account for the diagnosis of functional constipation.

7.5.2   Diarrhea

It is also difficult to define diarrhea. In addition to a higher frequency of defecation and an increased fecal output (more than 200 g per day), the Bristol stool form scale is used. In this scale consistency and shape of the stools are used to categorize the stools into one of seven types (Fig. 7.5).

Whereas constipation most often is caused by disordered motor function (of colon or pelvic floor), diarrhea is often the consequence of diminished resorption of water by the colonic mucosa. This can be caused by a variety of disorders such as inflammatory bowel disease (Crohn's disease and ulcerative colitis). Diarrhea can also be the consequence of malabsorption at the level of the small intestine, as for instance in celiac disease. Both in cases with acute and chronic diarrhea motility disorders should only be considered

Table 7.1 Characteristics of constipation

Low frequency of defecation (<3 week)
Necessity to strain excessively during defecation
Hard stools
Feeling of incomplete evacuation
Feeling of anorectal obstruction or blockade
Need for manual assistance during defecation

Bristol Stool Chart

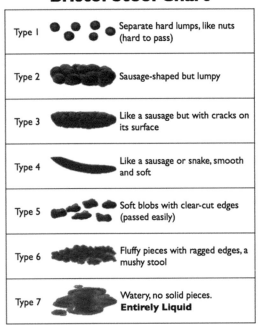

Type 1	Separate hard lumps, like nuts (hard to pass)
Type 2	Sausage-shaped but lumpy
Type 3	Like a sausage but with cracks on its surface
Type 4	Like a sausage or snake, smooth and soft
Type 5	Soft blobs with clear-cut edges (passed easily)
Type 6	Fluffy pieces with ragged edges, a mushy stool
Type 7	Watery, no solid pieces. **Entirely Liquid**

Fig. 7.5 Bristol stool scale. Stools are categorized based on consistency and form

when all other causes of diarrhea have been excluded (Table 7.2).

7.5.3 Distended Abdomen

Not infrequently the gastroenterologist sees patients whose predominant complaint is that they have a distended abdomen. Some of these patients do not really have abdominal distension but they perceive a feeling of bloating. In others the abdomen is visibly distended. This condition can be caused by serious conditions such as ascites, hepatosplenomegaly, and large tumors or cysts in the abdomen, but often the distension is brought about by accumulation of gas, fluid, or feces in the gastrointestinal tract, in particular in the colon. Such accumulation of liquid, gaseous, or solid material in the colon can take place when the colonic transit is slow.

It is also possible however to have a visibly distended abdomen in the absence of an increase of the contents of the abdomen. This is brought about by a combination of a low position of the

Table 7.2 Causes of diarrhea

| Osmotic diarrhea |
| Carbohydrate malabsorption |
| Lactase deficiency |
| Excessive intake of poorly absorbable carbohydrates (fructose, sorbitol) |
| Use or abuse of osmotic laxatives |
| Fat maldigestion and fat malabsorption |
| Other malabsorption syndromes |
| Bacterial overgrowth of small bowel |
| Secretory diarrhea |
| Infections |
| Bacterial |
| Parasites |
| Viral |
| Neuroendocrine tumors |
| Carcinoid |
| Medullary thyroid carcinoma |
| VIPoma |
| Inflammation of mucosa |
| Crohn's disease |
| Collagenous colitis |
| Ulcerative colitis |
| Celiac disease |
| Short bowel syndrome |
| Diarrhea mediated by abnormal motility |
| Hyperthyroidism |
| Carcinoid |
| Post-vagotomy |
| Irritable bowel syndrome |
| Diabetes mellitus |
| Intestinal pseudo-obstruction syndromes |
| Stimulant laxatives |

diaphragm, which is abnormally contracted, and relaxation of the abdominal wall muscles. Especially in patients with functional bowel disorders (such as irritable bowel syndrome) who complain of intermittent abdominal distension, this mechanism is frequently present.

7.5.4 Abdominal Pain

Pain in the abdomen can be caused by abnormal colonic motility in two ways. In patients with IBS-C abnormally strong contractions ("spasms") in a hypercontractile colon can lead to crampy

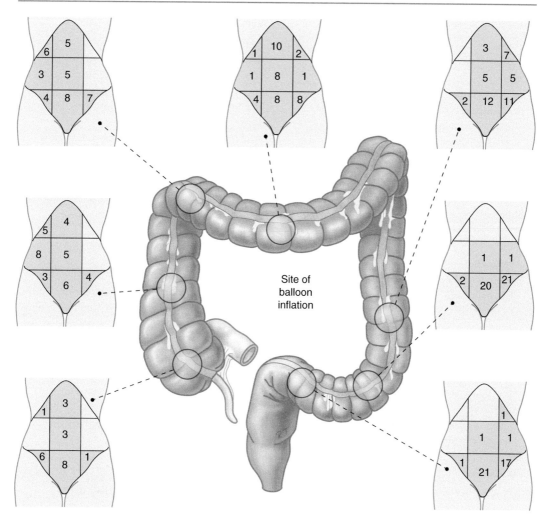

Fig. 7.6 Relationship between site of inflation of an intracolonic balloon and site of perception in 48 patients with abdominal pain. Note that the distension stimulus can be felt at areas of the abdomen that are rather remote from the position of the balloon (Published with kind permission of © Rogier Trompert Medical Art 2015)

pain. In patients with a hypocontractile colon accumulation of feces and gas can bring about abdominal discomfort and pain. It has been shown that the localization of pain that originates in the colon is not very precise. For instance, distension of the colon by inflation of a balloon in the ascending colon can lead to pain in the left lower quadrant (Fig. 7.6).

Some patients with constipation present with pain in the upper abdomen. Understandably the cause of the pain is then sought in the stomach and adjacent organs. Treatment of the constipation may alleviate the upper abdominal pain. Even when the pain in the upper abdomen

increases after meals, the colon may be the culprit. It is likely that the gastrocolonic response is involved in this postprandial increase of the pain.

7.6   Causes of Constipation

Constipation can have a variety of causes (Table 7.3).

Firstly, constipation can be the consequence of abnormal lifestyle and dietary habits. A diet that is extremely low in indigestible fiber and physical inactivity may promote constipation. When a subject repeatedly fails to respond to the

Table 7.3 Causes of constipation

| Lifestyle and dietary habits |
| Organic diseases |
| Drugs |
| Disordered function of colon and/or pelvic floor |
| Irritable bowel syndrome |
| Functional constipation |
| Pelvic floor dyssynergia (anismus) |

Table 7.4 Organic disorders that can be associated with constipation

| Mechanical obstruction |
| Carcinoma |
| Stricture |
| Enterocele |
| Metabolic diseases |
| Hypothyroidism |
| Diabetes mellitus |
| Disorders leading to muscular dysfunction |
| Amyloidosis |
| Scleroderma |
| Disorders leading to neuronal dysfunction |
| Hirschsprung's disease |
| Spinal cord lesions |
| Parkinson's disease |
| Multiple sclerosis |
| Miscellaneous |
| Depression |

Table 7.5 Drugs associated with constipation

Opioids	Morphine
Anticholinergic agents	Scopolamine (hyoscine)
Tricyclic antidepressants	Amitriptyline, nortriptyline
Calcium channel blockers	Nifedipine
Antiparkinson drugs	Amantadine
Sympathicomimetic agents	Ephedrine, terbutaline
Antipsychotic drugs	Chlorpromazine
Diuretics	Furosemide
Antihistaminics	Dexchlorpheniramine
Iron supplementation	Ferrous fumarate
Antacids, in particular calcium containing	
Antidiarrheal agents	loperamide

drugs, but the consequence of disordered function. The three most important functional disorders associated with constipation are:

1. Irritable bowel syndrome
2. Functional constipation
3. Pelvic floor dyssynergia (anismus)

The last-mentioned disorder will be discussed in Chap. 8.

7.6.1 Irritable Bowel Syndrome

Irritable bowel syndrome (IBS) is one of the most commonly encountered disorders in the daily practice of gastroenterologists and internists, as well as in general practice. The syndrome is characterized by abdominal pain accompanied by constipation, diarrhea, or an alternating pattern of constipation and diarrhea, in the absence of an organic cause.

The location of the pain in the abdomen is variable, but the left lower quadrant is most often the site that the patient points at, when asked to indicate the most painful area. Pain that shifts from one site to another is also common. Quite often patients have noticed that their pain diminishes after defecation. Another characteristic of the abdominal pain in IBS is that it increases at times when there is a change in bowel habits (change in frequency of defecation or change in

feeling of having to defecate, colonic contents may harden so much that evacuation of the rectum becomes difficult.

All organic diseases that result in a structural or functional narrowing of the lumen of the colon may lead to constipation (Table 7.4). Examples are colon cancer, complicated diverticular disease, and stricturing Crohn's disease.

Furthermore, disorders leading to damage to the neuronal systems that control colonic motility can lead to constipation. Examples of this are diabetes mellitus (with autonomic neuropathy), multiple sclerosis, and spinal cord lesions. Yet another group of causes of constipation is formed by drugs that inhibit colonic motility. These are listed in Table 7.5.

In many cases, however, constipation is not secondary to another disorder, another disease, or form of the stools). In the Rome III criteria for IBS, these three characteristics are included as features that lend support to the diagnosis. In addition to characteristics described above, there are symptoms that further support the diagnosis of IBS, such as an abnormally low or high frequency of defecation, an abnormal consistency of the feces, disordered defecation, mucus excretion, and distension of the abdomen or feeling of distension. The Rome III criteria for IBS are summarized in Table 7.6.

IBS can be present and have its onset at any age, but the prevalence is highest at young adolescent age (Fig. 7.7). The disorder is diagnosed

more often in women than in men (ratio approximately 1.5:1).

Four subtypes of IBS can be distinguished on the basis of the form and consistency of the patient's stools as scored with the Bristol stool scale (Fig. 7.5). These are IBS with constipation (IBS-C), IBS with diarrhea (IBS-D), mixed IBS (IBS-M), and unsubtyped IBS. The criteria for the IBS subtypes are listed in Table 7.7 and graphically displayed in Fig. 7.8.

The most frequently reported motor abnormality in patients with constipation-predominant IBS (IBS-C) is an increased frequency of haustrating colonic contractions. X-ray examination and endoscopy may show hyperhaustration, especially in the sigmoid colon. These findings are by no means of diagnostic value, since the overlap with findings in healthy subjects is large. Increased motility in constipated patients seems to be paradoxical. However, it should be borne in mind that the contractions of the colon are largely non-propulsive; they can lead to stagnation rather

Table 7.6   Rome III criteria for IBS

Recurrent abdominal pain or discomfort, at least 3 days per month in the last 3 months, associated with two or more of the following:
1. Improvement with defecation
2. Onset associated with a change in frequency of stool
3. Onset associated with a change in form (appearance) of stool
These criteria must have been fulfilled for the last 3 months, and symptom onset must have been at least 6 months prior to diagnosis
Supportive symptoms that are not part of the diagnostic criteria include:
Abnormal stool frequency (>3 bowel movements per day or <3 per week)
Abnormal stool form (lumpy/hard or loose/watery stool)
Defecation straining
Urgency
Feeling of incomplete bowel movement
Passing mucus
Bloating

Table 7.7   Definitions of IBS subtypes

IBS with constipation (IBS-C)
$\geq$25 % hard or lumpy stools (Bristol 1 or 2)
<25 % loose or watery stools (Bristol 6 or 7)
IBS with diarrhea (IBS-D)
$\geq$25 % loose or watery stools (Bristol 6 or 7)
<25 % hard or lumpy stools (Bristol 1 or 2)
Mixed IBS (IBS-M)
$\geq$25 % hard or lumpy stools (Bristol 1 or 2)
$\geq$25 % loose or watery stools (Bristol 6 or 7)
Unsubtyped IBS
Insufficient abnormality of stool consistency to meet criteria for IBS-C, IBS-D, or IBS-M

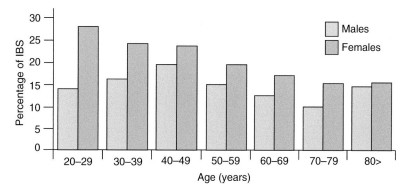

Fig. 7.7   Prevalence of IBS

Fig. 7.8 Categorization of IBS patients into IBS-C, IBS-D, IBS-M, and unsubtyped IBS

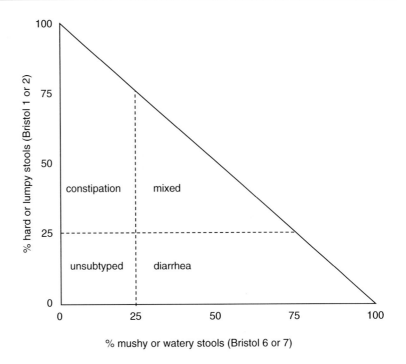

Fig. 7.9 IBS patients experience pain in the colon at lower balloon distension volumes than healthy controls

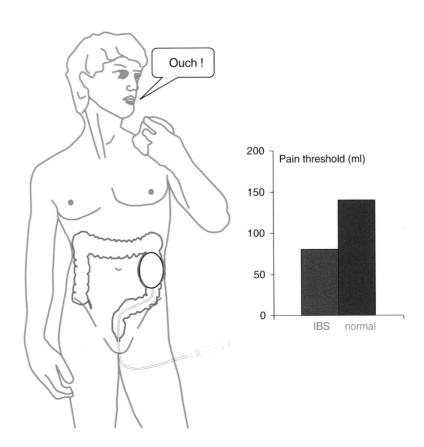

than transit. Another finding in patients with IBS with constipation (IBS-C) is a decreased incidence of mass movements. It has also been reported that patients with IBS have an exaggerated gastrocolonic response. This might explain the postprandial increase in abdominal pain reported by a subset of patients with IBS.

In all subtypes of IBS hypersensitivity of the colon plays an important role in the generation of symptoms. Studies have shown that the threshold for perception of visceral stimuli (e.g., balloon distension) is lowered in patients with IBS (Fig. 7.9). The tolerance for somatic stimuli (e.g., submersion of the hand in ice water) is not different from that in healthy control subjects (Fig. 7.10).

7.6.2   Functional Constipation

According to the Rome III criteria the diagnosis of functional constipation can be made when two or more symptoms of constipation are present (see Table 7.1), when the patient rarely has loose or watery stools when no laxatives are used, and when there are insufficient criteria for IBS (Table 7.8). Scientific studies have shown that

Table 7.8   Rome III criteria for functional constipation

1. Must include two or more of the following:
(a) Straining during at least 25 % of defecations
(b) Lumpy or hard stools in at least 25 % of defecations
(c) Sensation of incomplete evacuation for at least 25 % of defecations
(d) Sensation of anorectal obstruction/blockage for at least 25 % of defecations
(e) Manual maneuvers to facilitate at least 25 % of defecations (e.g., digital evacuation, support of the pelvic floor)
(f) Fewer than three defecations per week
2. Loose stools are rarely present without the use of laxatives
3. There are insufficient criteria for IBS

Criteria must have been fulfilled for the last 3 months, and symptom onset must be at least 6 months prior to diagnosis

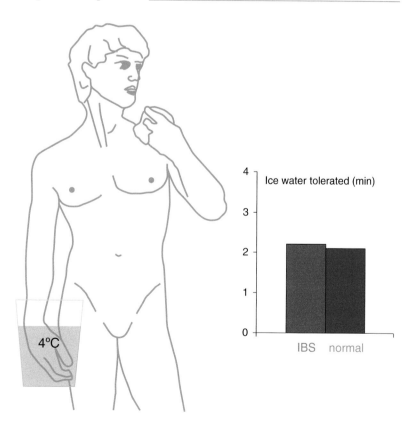

Fig. 7.10   IBS patients do not have a lower perception threshold for somatic pain stimuli, such as elicited by submersion of the hand in ice water

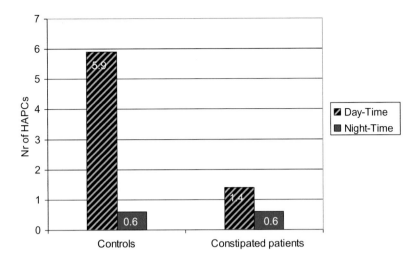

Fig. 7.11 Decreased number of HAPCs in patients with constipation

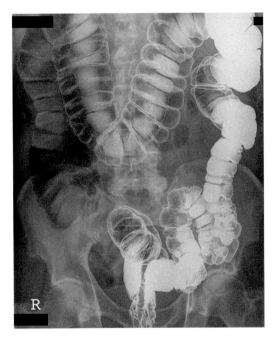

Fig. 7.12 Elongation of the colon in a patient with constipation

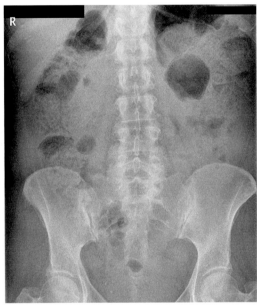

Fig. 7.13 Plain abdominal X-ray showing fecal stasis

patients with functional constipation, on average, have diminished colonic motility: the incidence of both the haustrating and the mass contractions is decreased (Fig. 7.11). When the constipation is severe, the term "colonic inertia" ("lazy colon") is sometimes used to denote this condition. Not infrequently patients with severe functional constipation have an abnormally long and abnormally wide colon, sometimes with decreased

haustration. This can be seen on a barium enema radiograph or endoscopically (Fig. 7.12). A plain abdominal X-ray may show increased opacification by fecal material, indicative of fecal stasis (Fig. 7.13).

At microscopic examination of the colon of patients with functional constipation (acquired post-mortem or surgically), a decreased number of neurons in the intramural plexuses in the colon or a decreased number of interstitial cells of Cajal can be found. It is unclear however whether these alterations are cause or consequence of many years of severe constipation and colonic distension.

7.6.3 Ogilvie's Syndrome

Ogilvie's syndrome is a relatively rare acute form of colonic atony. It is characterized by non-passage of feces and extreme distension of the entire colon with air/gas. The syndrome occurs mostly in elderly subjects, often during the course of a severe illness or postoperatively. The cause of the syndrome is unknown, but it is clear that a decreased tone of colonic smooth muscle plays an important role. When left untreated, perforation ("blow-out") of the colon, mostly at the level of the cecum, can occur. One of the possible interventions is decompression by means of colonoscopic desufflation. However, the effect of desufflation is often short-lived. Drug treatment is also possible. Intravenous administration of neostigmine, an acetylcholinesterase inhibitor, often leads to immediate restoration of colonic tone. Because the drug can cause severe bradycardia and asystole, it has to be administered under electrocardiographic monitoring. The oral acetylcholinesterase inhibitor pyridostigmine can also be used to treat Ogilvie's syndrome. Sometimes colectomy has to be performed.

7.7 Treatment of Irritable Bowel Syndrome and Functional Constipation

7.7.1 Treatment of Irritable Bowel Syndrome

In the management of IBS, explanation about the condition is of paramount importance. Merely informing the patient that no organic cause of the symptoms can be found does not have a sufficiently beneficial effect. Information about the pathogenesis of IBS obtained in scientific studies, although not translatable to diagnostic tests, can be shared with the patient. Factors such as hyperperception of visceral stimuli, disordered gut motility, and abnormal bacterial flora can be brought into the equation. Many patients can cope with the symptoms better when they know what causes them.

Experts' opinion on the use of a fiber-enriched diet in the management of IBS has evolved notably during the past decennia. During the 1970s, a fiber-rich diet became viewed upon as healthy on the basis of epidemiological observations. In particular for IBS a diet as rich as possible in dietary fiber became the most important therapeutic option. A fiber-rich diet decreases constipation in IBS-C. However, it is now clear that, in IBS, coarse insoluble dietary fibers such as in bran can lead to an increase in pain. Soluble fibers such as in the bulk-forming agents psyllium seed husk (Metamucil®) or sterculia gum (karaya gum) do not increase pain and thus are to be preferred. Soluble fibers can also have a beneficial effect in patients with IBS-D and IBS-M because they tend to make loose stools less loose and to diminish the fluctuations in stool consistency.

In patients with IBS-C not only soluble fiber but also other laxatives, in particular osmotically active agents, can be used. These will be discussed in Sect. 7.7.2. In IBS patients in whom diarrhea is a prominent symptom, loperamide may help to increase the consistency of the stools.

When spasms of colonic smooth muscle are thought to play a role, spasmolytic drugs may be attempted. These drugs (e.g., mebeverine and otilonium bromide) act in part by a direct effect on calcium influx in the smooth muscle cells and in part by an antimuscarinic effect. Peppermint oil also has spasmolytic effects, which appear to be mediated by a local action on calcium influx.

Paracetamol can be used to diminish pain in IBS, although the effect of this drug on IBS-related pain is often described as disappointing. NSAIDs and opiates seem to be more effective, but their side effects limit widespread use in IBS.

In IBS patients in whom abdominal pain is severe and other measures fail to bring adequate relief, a tricyclic antidepressant can be used. The agent that was best studied in IBS is amitriptyline. Several studies have shown that this drug increases the threshold for perception and pain of intestinal stimuli. Usually a low dose (10–25 mg at night time) is used for this application. The drug is taken at night time because the most frequent side effect is drowsiness. When prescribing the drug it is important to explain to the patient that the aim is not to treat depression but to decrease visceral hyperperception. Treatment must be continued for at least 6 weeks before conclusions regarding its effectiveness can be drawn. When a tricyclic antidepressant is not tolerated or is not sufficiently effective or when its constipating features are undesirable, a selective serotonin reuptake inhibitor (SSRI), such as citalopram, 10–20 mg once daily, can be tried.

There is conflicting information about the effectiveness of probiotics. Meta-analyses show a very modest superiority over placebo, but it is yet unclear which microorganism or combinations of microorganisms are to be preferred.

Rifaximin is a poorly absorbed antibiotic that was shown to reduce symptoms and improve well-being in patients with IBS. Its use is based on the hypothesis that bacterial overgrowth is an important pathogenetic factor in IBS. There is no consensus on this concept.

Linaclotide is a guanylate cyclase inhibitor that increases net water secretion by the gut, thus reducing constipation. In addition, this locally active drug also has an effect on visceral pain. It has been shown to be effective in patients with IBS-C.

The prostaglandin analogue lubiprostone promotes colonic chloride secretion and motility, thereby reducing constipation and pain in patients with IBC-C. It is not marketed yet in most European countries.

The effect of hypnotherapy on symptoms and bowel function in IBS has been studied quite extensively. The results of these studies indicate that this treatment is more effective than standard care with comparable levels of patient-care provider contact.

7.7.2 Treatment of Functional Constipation

The first step in the management of functional constipation is to evaluate whether constipation-promoting factors are present, such as drugs, limited mobility, or a low-fiber diet. When these factors have been eliminated and constipation persists, the next step in the treatment comprises prescribing osmotic laxatives and/or bulk-forming agents.

Osmotically active laxatives work by preventing the reabsorption of water by the colon, making the stools more loose. They do not have a direct stimulatory effect on colonic motility.

Nowadays, probably the most popular laxatives within the group of osmotically active agents are several forms of polyethylene glycol, also known as macrogol. All of these are to be taken in liquid form, dissolved in water. Since macrogols are not absorbed, there are practically no side effects.

Another possibility is to use magnesium oxide or magnesium hydroxide, which are available in tablet form. In patients with a normal renal function there is no increase in serum magnesium levels, but in patients with renal insufficiency care must be taken to avoid hypermagnesemia. Other osmotically active salts, such as magnesium sulfate, sodium sulfate, and sodium phosphate, have more potential side effects.

The synthetic disaccharide lactulose is also a popular laxative. Lactulose is osmotically active, but in addition it provides the colonic bacterial flora with a substrate, and some of the formed breakdown products stimulate colonic motility and transit. A disadvantage of lactulose can be that it leads to increased production of gas in the colon, which limits its use in patients in whom bloating is often already a bothersome symptom.

When the abovementioned measures are not sufficiently effective, so-called contact laxatives can be used. To this group belong bisacodyl, picosulfate, and sennosides (Fig. 7.14). These drugs act by direct stimulation of the colon, hence the name contact laxatives. Their precise mode of action is unknown.

There are also systemically active drugs that stimulate colonic motility via a systemic mode of action. Prucalopride, a new 5-HT$_4$-serotonin agonist, has been shown to be effective in constipation that does not respond sufficiently to laxatives. Lubiprostone, a prostaglandin derivative, stimu-

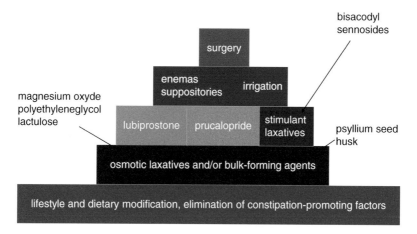

Fig. 7.14 Stepwise approach of strategies in the treatment of functional constipation

lates intestinal secretion which softens the stools and promotes bowel movement. The acetylcholinesterase inhibitor pyridostigmine, used by neurologists to treat myasthenia gravis, can also be used – off label – to treat therapy-refractory constipation, but may be accompanied by cholinergic side effects.

Another option is to stimulate colonic motility by means of an enema. Enemas may contain osmotic laxatives or a stimulant laxative, or both, or may consist of water or saline solution only.

Sacral nerve stimulation is a treatment modality that was initially developed for fecal incontinence, but in recent years its application in severe constipation has also been studied. After a trial period with an external stimulator, responsive patients are fitted with an implantable device (Fig. 7.15). So far, studies on the efficacy of sacral nerve stimulation in constipation have yielded conflicting results. Use of the technique outside research settings cannot yet be advised. It appears likely that the influence of sacral nerve stimulation on anorectal function also involves stimulation of afferent pathways.

In highly exceptional cases, resection of the colon is carried out to treat severe, therapy-resistant constipation. Experience has taught us that resection of parts of the colon only has a temporary effect on the pattern of defecation. Most experts would agree that subtotal colec-

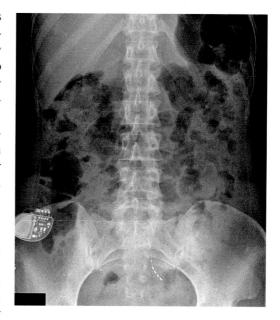

Fig. 7.15 Implanted stimulator and electrode lead for sacral nerve stimulation in a patient with severe functional constipation

tomy with ileorectal anastomosis is the procedure of choice, although the long-term outcome remains difficult to predict. Alternatively an end ileostomy can be constructed. In cases when colectomy is performed and continuity is restored, presence of defecation disorders should be excluded preoperatively with balloon expulsion testing and defecography.

Anorectum

8

8.1 Introduction

The last parts of the gastrointestinal canal, the rectum and the anus, take care of a number of specialized functions. These are to retain the produced feces until a suitable moment for defecation has arrived and, subsequently, to achieve effective expulsion of the fecal mass. The rectum and the anal sphincter exert these functions in close collaboration with the pelvic floor. Thus, smooth muscle (rectal muscles and internal anal sphincter [IAS]) and striated muscle (pelvic floor and external anal sphincter [EAS]) work closely together in this area. Disordered functioning of the anus, rectum, and pelvic floor can result in two groups of functional problems: impaired defecation and fecal incontinence.

8.2 Anatomy

The rectum, 10–15 cm in length, is the most distal part of the colon. This is an extraperitoneally located part of the gastrointestinal canal. The longitudinal muscles of the rectum are continuous with the longitudinal muscles of the colon. At the transition from the sigmoid colon to the rectum, the three longitudinal taeniae join to form the continuous longitudinal layer of the rectum. The internal anal sphincter (IAS), 2–3 cm long, is continuous with the circular muscles of the rectum. Its smooth muscle is not under voluntary control.

The external anal sphincter (EAS), 3–4 cm long, surrounds the IAS. The EAS is a striated muscle sphincter that is under voluntary control. This sphincter collaborates closely with the pelvic floor, a structure composed of number of striated muscles. In the direct surroundings of the anus, the most important muscles of the pelvic floor are the puborectalis muscle and the levator ani muscle. The puborectalis muscle is U-shaped and forms a sling around the distal part of the rectum. Its two anterior ends are inserted into the pubic bone. The puborectalis continuously pulls the rectum forward and creates a sharp angle between the rectal and the anal canal (Fig. 8.1). The tonic contraction of the levator ani muscle maintains an elevated position of the pelvic floor and the anus. During defecation the levator ani muscle and the puborectalis muscle relax, leading to a downward displacement of the pelvic floor, as well as to a more obtuse anorectal angle.

The innervation of anus and rectum is complex. Like elsewhere in the gastrointestinal canal, the rectum has a myenteric and submucosal plexus. The extrinsic innervation of the IAS is supplied by the autonomic nervous system (sympathetic and parasympathetic). The sympathetic fibers originate in the L5 segment of the spinal cord and reach the IAS via the hypogastric plexus and the pelvic plexus. The parasympathetic fibers leave the spinal cord in the segments S2 to S4 and they reach the IAS via the pelvic plexus. The innervation of the EAS is via the pudendal nerve

© Springer International Publishing Switzerland 2016
A.J. Bredenoord et al., *A Guide to Gastrointestinal Motility Disorders*,
DOI 10.1007/978-3-319-26938-2_8

91

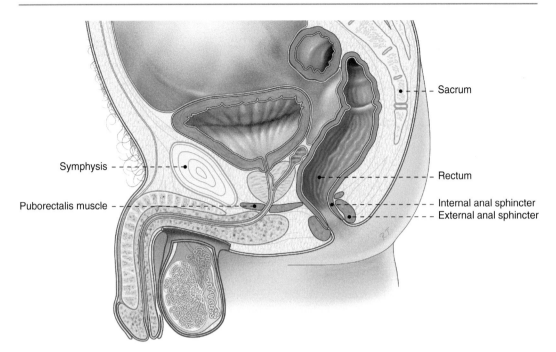

Fig. 8.1 Anatomy of the pelvic floor and surrounding structures (Published with kind permission of © Rogier Trompert Medical Art 2015)

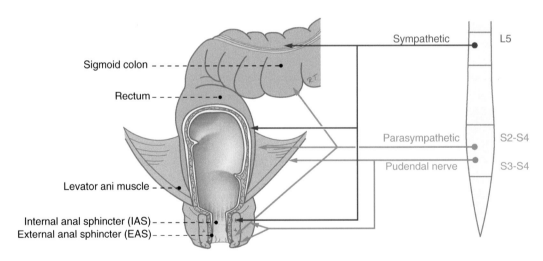

Fig. 8.2 Nerve supply to the rectum, anus, and pelvic floor (Published with kind permission of © Rogier Trompert Medical Art 2015)

that comes from the sacral part of the spinal cord. The pelvic floor muscles also receive neuronal input via this nerve (Fig. 8.2).

In addition to this efferent, motility-driving innervation, there is an important afferent neuronal circuitry in the rectoanal area. Its function is to relay information from the sensory elements in the wall of the rectum and anus to the enteric nervous system but also to the brain. The system makes it possible to feel the urge to defecate, and the combination of sensory information from the anal canal and the rectum even makes it possible to perceive whether the contents of the rectum are solid, liquid, or gaseous.

8.3 Anorectal Constipation

As discussed in Chap. 7, constipation is often caused by disordered colon function. However, in a subset of patients with constipation, the cause of the constipation lies in abnormal function or an anatomical abnormality in the anorectal area, including the pelvic floor.

8.3.1 How to Recognize Constipation Caused by an Anorectal Disorder

The patient's history can provide important information that may help to distinguish between constipation caused by disordered colonic function and constipation caused by an abnormality in the anorectal area. When the patient reports that he or she rarely experiences an urge to defecate but that when the urge occurs it is not a major problem to empty the bowel, it is not likely that the cause of the constipation can be found in the anorectum or the pelvic floor. On the other hand, if the patient regularly experiences the urge to defecate but is then unable to expel the feces, the possibility of an anorectal disorder must be considered. Furthermore, a sudden onset of the constipation and a young age at the onset of the constipation point in the direction of an anorectal disorder.

However, it can be difficult to differentiate between the two types of defecation on the basis of the history. Many patients with colonic constipation have hard stools, which can be difficult to evacuate, even when the pelvic floor and the anorectum function normally.

8.3.1.1 Colonic Transit Tests

Some clinicians use a colonic transit test to distinguish constipation based on an anorectal disorder from constipation caused by a colonic function disorder. When the holdup of the markers (radioopaque pellets or radioactivity) is in the proximal colon, this would favor a diagnosis of a colonic dysfunction, whereas stasis in the rectosigmoid area would support a diagnosis of dyssynergic defecation. However, there is no evidence that corroborates this view. On the other hand, a study in healthy subjects has shown that voluntary suppression of defecation, which mimics a defecation disorder, leads to stasis of the markers in the right colon in a proportion of the individuals. This suggests that colonic transit tests do not provide reliable information as to the mechanism of the constipation. A colonic transit test is thus not recommended for distinguishing between functional constipation and dyssynergic defecation.

8.3.2 Functional and Structural Causes

Defecation disorders can be caused by various abnormalities. Two groups of causes can be distinguished. Firstly, there may be abnormal function of the anal sphincter or the pelvic floor muscles. This can occur in a behavioral abnormality known as dyssynergic defecation and in Hirschsprung's disease. On the other hand, disordered rectal evacuation can also be caused by a structural abnormality that leads to obstruction. In the next paragraphs the functional and structural abnormalities that can lead disordered defecation will be discussed.

8.4 Constipation Caused by Disordered Anorectal Function

8.4.1 Dyssynergic Defecation

In patients with dyssynergic defecation, the pelvic floor and the EAS do not relax sufficiently during attempts to defecate. In many cases, these muscles even contract paradoxically. Other names that have been given to this disorder are spastic pelvic floor syndrome and anismus. Dyssynergic defecation is an acquired condition that can have its debut at any age but often starts in adolescence. Not infrequently, psychological factors play a role. Dyssynergic defecation has been shown to be associated with sexual abuse.

8.4.2 Diagnosis

The diagnosis of dyssynergic defecation requires specialized tests. Some claim that the diagnosis can be made with digital examination, but this view is not shared by many experts in the field.

A useful technique for assessment of pelvic floor function is defecography. In this procedure videofluorography is used to visualize the defecation process. The rectum is filled with a thickened barium suspension, the vagina is filled with contrast, and the small bowel is made radioopaque with orally ingested contrast. Using laterolateral X-ray, moving images of the pelvic region of the patient – who is seated on a toilet – are obtained. After having acquired images in rest and during straining, the patient is instructed to empty the rectum. In the analysis of the acquired images, attention is paid to the patient's ability to empty the rectum, to the widening of the rectoanal angle, and to anatomical abnormalities that can occur during straining (Fig. 8.3). Nowadays, defecography can also be carried out with magnetic resonance imaging (MRI) (Fig. 8.4). The

advantage over radiography is that no ionizing radiation is applied. The disadvantage is that the investigation can only be carried out with the patient in a supine position.

In addition to defecography also the balloon expulsion test, rectoanal manometry, and electromyography can be used to diagnose dyssynergic defecation. In the balloon expulsion test, the patient is requested to expel a balloon that was inserted into the rectum and then inflated. Patients with dyssynergic defecation have difficulty evacuating the balloon.

Electromyography of the EAS can be carried out with needle electrodes, with skin electrodes, or with electrodes mounted on anal plug. The electromyographical hallmark of the dyssynergic defecation is a paradoxical increase of EAS activity during attempts to defecate (Fig. 8.5). The key finding in rectoanal manometry is the absence of a fall in sphincter pressure during attempts to defecate. The sphincter pressure may even increase rather than decrease (Fig. 8.6). It has been argued that balloon expulsion test, manometry, and electromyography are prone to lead to false-positive

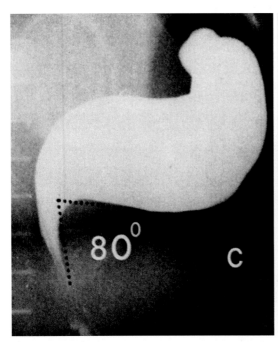
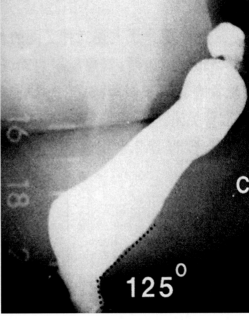

Fig. 8.3 Conventional defecography (using X-ray) in a healthy subject. Lateral views, right-hand side is posterior. *Left panel*: in rest. *Right panel*: during defecation. During defecation the rectoanal angle, brought about by the puborectalis muscle, becomes more obtuse

results because the patient is likely to be reluctant to perform a defecation-like maneuver in an nonphysiological position with an investigator in the immediate vicinity. Therefore, in many centers defecography is the preferred test for spastic pelvic floor syndrome.

The Rome III criteria for dyssynergic defecation are listed in Table 8.1.

8.4.3 Treatment

In the treatment of dyssynergic defecation, biofeedback training plays a pivotal role. In this therapy the patient is taught to relax the EAS and the pelvic floor during defecation attempts. To achieve this, a manometric or EMG signal is recorded from the EAS and visualized for the patient. The patient is instructed to diminish EAS activity during attempted defecation. This type of training is provided by specialized physiotherapists. If treatment is successful, dyssynergic def-

ecation can be cured, but failures and relapses do occur.

Experience with treatment of the condition with botulinum toxin injection in the EAS is limited. At best a short-lived effect is obtained. Surgical treatment of dyssynergic defecation, such as EAS sphincterotomy, has been found to be unsuccessful and is not recommended.

8.4.4 Hirschsprung's Disease

Hirschsprung's disease is a congenital disorder in which nerve cells are absent in a part of the distal colon. During normal fetal development, cells from the neural crest migrate into the colon to form the intramural plexuses. In Hirschsprung's disease, the migration is not complete and part of the colon lacks the ganglion cells that normally regulate the activity of the colon. The affected segment of the colon cannot relax, thus creating an obstruction. The aganglionic segment of the

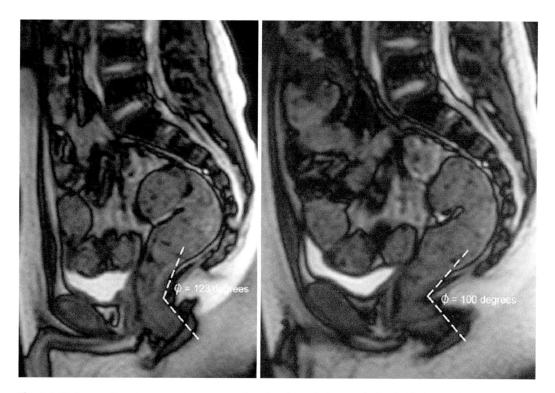

Fig. 8.4 Defecography using magnetic resonance imaging. Lateral views, right-hand side is posterior. *Left panel*: in rest. *Right panel*: during defecation

Fig. 8.5 Electromyography
of the external anal sphincter
(EAS). *Upper panel*: healthy
subject. During straining as if
defecating there is a decrease
in EMG activity. *Lower panel*:
patient with anismus. The
EMG activity increases during
attempted defecation

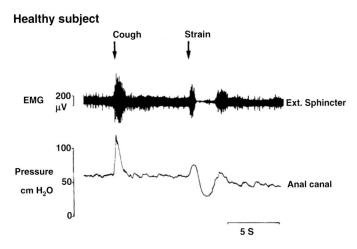

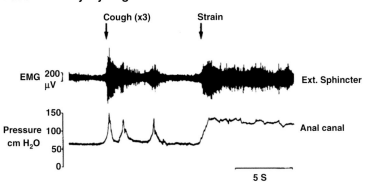

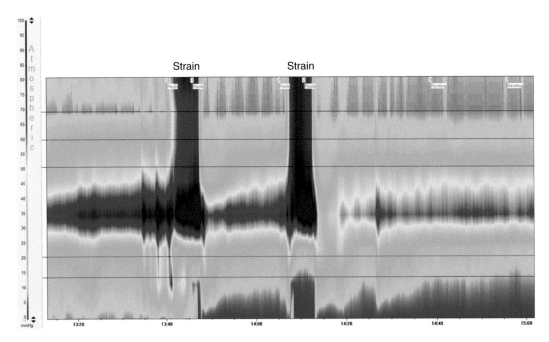

Fig. 8.6 High-resolution manometry of anorectum in a patient with dyssynergic defecation. During attempts to simu-
lated defecation (indicated with "strain"), there is an increase in sphincter pressure, rather than a decrease

Table 8.1   Rome III criteria for dyssynergic defecation

1. The patient must satisfy diagnostic criteria for functional constipation
2. During repeated attempts to defecate must have *at least 2* of the following:
(a) Evidence of impaired evacuation, based on balloon expulsion test or imaging
(b) Inappropriate contraction of the pelvic floor muscles (i.e., anal sphincter or puborectalis) or less than 20 % relaxation of basal resting sphincter pressure by manometry, imaging, or EMG
Criteria fulfilled for the last 3 months with symptom onset at least 6 months prior to diagnosis

colon always involves most distal end, but its length is variable. The severity of the constipation depends on the length of the affected segment.

In most cases, Hirschsprung's disease leads to severe constipation from birth onward and the diagnosis is usually made in the first year of life. In rare cases, when the length of the affected segment is very short, the diagnosis is not made until adulthood.

8.4.4.1 Diagnosis

In the diagnosis of Hirschsprung's disease, rectoanal manometry plays an important role. The characteristic abnormality is absence of the so-called rectoanal inhibition reflex. This reflex is elicited by distension of the rectum, by inflating a balloon, and the normal response to this distension is relaxation of the IAS. In patients with Hirschsprung's disease, the IAS does not relax, due to the absence of ganglion cells in the rectum. The diagnosis is confirmed by histological examination of deep biopsies taken from the rectum. Alternatively, more superficial, mucosal biopsies can be taken and stained for acetylcholinesterase. This will show an increased number of axons that have grown in from other areas ("axonal sprouting").

8.4.4.2 Treatment

The treatment of Hirschsprung's disease is surgical. The essence of the operation is that the aganglionic part of the colon is removed and the continuity is restored, with preservation of the sphincter complex. Nowadays this is usually done with a combination of laparoscopy and transanal approach.

8.5 Constipation Caused by Structural Abnormalities in the Anorectal Region

Any alteration in the anatomy of the anorectum that leads to a stenosis can cause constipation. The rectum can become narrowed by malignant tumors, such as a carcinoma. It is obvious that in middle-aged and elderly patients presenting with sudden-onset constipation, a tumor must be excluded as soon as possible, before other diagnostic tests into the cause of the constipation are initiated.

Apart from tumors, benign anatomical alterations in the anorectal area can lead to constipation. One of these is the enterocele. This is a herniation of small intestinal loop in the space between the vagina and rectum. The enterocele can obstruct the rectum and thus lead to a defecation disorder that is clinically indistinguishable from dyssynergic defecation. The abnormality is seen more often in women, in particular after hysterectomy. For the diagnosis of enterocele, defecography is the method of choice. This requires additional opacification of the small intestine so that the small bowel loop that descends into the rectovaginal septum is visualized (Fig. 8.7). The diagnosis can also be made with MR defecography. Treatment of a symptomatic enterocele is surgical.

Another anatomical abnormality that can cause obstructed defecation is rectal intussusception. In this condition part of the rectal wall invaginates during straining. As with enterocele, the diagnosis is best made with defecography or MR defecography (Fig. 8.6). Intussusception can be corrected surgically, usually including fixation of the rectum to the sacrum (rectopexia). Because intussusception is often associated with dyssynergic defecation, it is advised to refer the patient for biofeedback training first.

A rectocele is a diverticulum-like bulging of the anterior rectal wall, into the direction of the vagina. Again, this abnormality is best diagnosed with defecography or MR defecography.

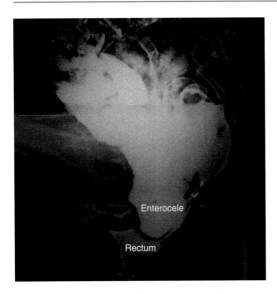

Fig. 8.7 Defecographic image showing enterocele. Lateral view, right-hand side is posterior

Small rectoceles, only seen during straining, are considered normal. In patients with large rectoceles, it is often uncertain whether the abnormality is the cause or the consequence of the constipation. Some patients with rectocele report that they can defecate better when they reduce the rectocele by applying pressure on the posterior wall of the vagina. The results of surgical treatment of rectocele are variable. This probably reflects the uncertain causal relationships between rectocele and constipation. As with enterocele, biofeedback training of the pelvic floor is recommended when there is suspicion of dyssynergic defecation.

8.6   Fecal Incontinence

Fecal incontinence is defined as unintended loss of rectal contents. Such unintended loss may be limited to flatus, or to liquid stools, or the incontinence may include loss of solid stools. In the mildest forms of fecal incontinence, the patient notices that traces of feces are present in the underwear (soiling) and occasionally control over gas and fluid feces is falling short. Mild forms of incontinence occur rather frequently, and the prevalence of mild incontinence increases with age. Patients with severe fecal incontinence also lose large amounts of formed stools. The social impact of fecal incontinence is often substantial.

8.6.1   Investigations in Incontinence

The history of patients with fecal incontinence often provides important clues as to the cause of the symptom. In particular information about difficult childbirth, trauma, or surgical procedures in the anal region and neurological abnormalities should be obtained. Inspection of the perianal region and digital examination of the rectum give information about sphincter symmetry, sphincter tone at rest and during squeezing, and absence of presence of mucosal prolapse.

Several additional tests can help to identify the cause of the incontinence (Fig. 8.8). Pressures in the anal sphincter complex can be studied with anorectal manometry. This test is always combined with sensitivity testing: the rectal balloon that is used to elicit the rectoanal inhibition reflex is also used to assess the perception of rectal distension stimuli. Assessment of sensitivity for electrical stimuli, measurement of pudendal nerve motor latency, and electromyography of the EAS are used in specialized centers only. Anal intraluminal ultrasound imaging provides important information on the integrity of the EAS and the IAS (Fig. 8.9). It is often performed in the same session as anorectal manometry and distension testing.

8.6.2   Causes and Treatment of Fecal Incontinence

It is important to identify the cause of the fecal incontinence, because this determines the therapeutic options. The causes can be broadly divided into myogenic and neurogenic. Irrespective of the cause of the incontinence, the first approach can always be to optimize the pattern of defecation and the consistency of the stools, e.g., by using a bulk-forming agent or loperamide.

Fig. 8.8 Some of the tools used in rectoanal function studies. *From top to bottom*: balloon and catheter for manometry, elicitation of the rectoanal inhibition reflex and mechanosensitivity, catheter for electrosensitivity testing, catheter for measurement of pudendal nerve motor latency, probe for intraluminal ultrasonography

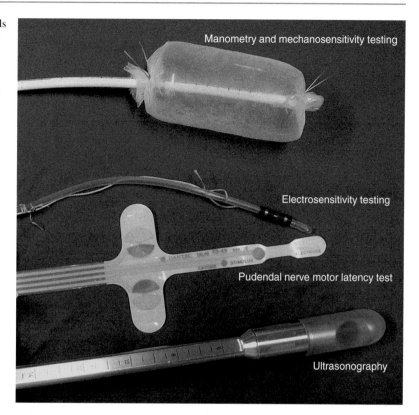

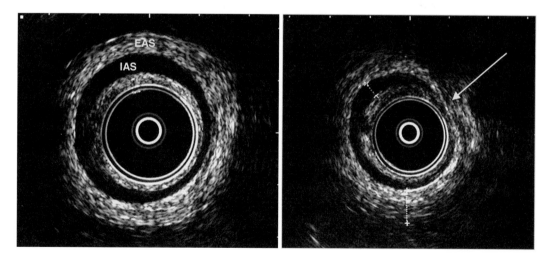

Fig. 8.9 Intraluminal ultrasound images of the anal sphincter complex. *Left panel*: normal. *Right panel*: anus with defects in IAS and EAS (indicated by *arrow*)

8.6.2.1 Myogenic Causes

Generalized loss of anal sphincter muscle tissue or localized sphincter tears (IAS, EAS, or both) can occur as a consequence of labor and delivery, by other trauma to the region, by surgical procedures in the area, or by neuromuscular disorders, such as myotonic dystrophia. Some forms of myogenic fecal incontinence can be treated surgically. Especially when there is a well-defined local defect in one or both of the sphincters, surgical sphincteroplasty is likely to lead to improvement.

8.6.2.2 Neurogenic Causes

Fecal incontinence can also be caused by degenerative or traumatic lesions to the nerves supplying the anorectal region. One of the best studied neurogenic causes is pudendal nerve injury, which may be caused by prolonged labor, by excessive straining in severe constipation, or by neuropathy, e.g., in diabetes mellitus.

When fecal incontinence has a neurogenic cause, treatment options are usually limited. The first approach must be sphincter training under the guidance of a specialized physiotherapist.

In patients who fail to respond to initial management, injection of an anal bulking agent, sacral nerve stimulation, and post-anal sphincter repair can be considered. The results are disappointing however. Dynamic graciloplasty and artificial anal sphincter devices are associated with significant morbidity and should still be considered experimental. Colostomy is the ultimate refuge.

8.7 Perianal and Rectoanal Pain

Pain in the anorectal region can be caused by an organic abnormality such as an abscess, a thrombosed hemorrhoid, or anorectal carcinoma. However, in a substantial proportion of patients with pain in this region, none of these abnormalities can be found and a functional disorder is considered.

8.7.1 Coccygodynia

Coccygodynia is characterized by chronic pain in the perineum and its surroundings. The pain is elicited or aggravated by touching the coccyx. The syndrome has an unknown etiology. Infiltration with a local analgesic or even coccygectomy is attempted in severe cases.

Table 8.2 Rome III criteria for the levator ani syndrome

Must include all of the following:
1. Chronic or recurrent rectal pain or aching
2. Episodes last at least 20 min
3. Exclusion of other causes of rectal pain such as ischemia, inflammatory bowel disease, cryptitis, intramuscular abscess and fissure, hemorrhoids, prostatitis, and coccygodynia
4. Tenderness during posterior traction on the puborectalis

8.7.2 Levator Ani Syndrome

The levator ani syndrome is characterized by chronic pain in the anorectal area, for which no explanation can be found. It is assumed that a high tone of the pelvic floor muscles plays a role. The Rome III criteria for the levator ani syndrome include that pain can be elicited or aggravated by posterior traction on the puborectalis muscle (Table 8.2).

Treatment of the levator ani syndrome is difficult. Biofeedback training, muscle-relaxing agents (such as diazepam), sitz baths, and botulinum toxin injections are sometimes advised, but evidence for the effectiveness of these treatment modalities is not available. Given the uncertainties regarding the etiology of the syndrome, surgical treatment (e.g., sphincterotomy) cannot be recommended.

8.7.3 Proctalgia Fugax

Proctalgia fugax is a rare syndrome characterized by short episodes of severe pain in the anal region with long symptom-free intervals. The pain is of such intensity that the patient has to abandon normal activities. Patient can be woken up during the night by a pain attack. The Rome III criteria for proctalgia fugax are listed in Table 8.3.

Table 8.3 Rome III criteria for proctalgia fugax

Must include all of the following:
1. Recurrent episodes of pain localized to the anus or lower rectum
2. Episodes last from seconds to minutes
3. There is no anorectal pain between episodes

The cause of proctalgia fugax is still unclear. It is assumed that spasm of the muscles in the rectum, in the anal sphincter, or in the pelvic floor plays a role. Some families with a hereditary form of proctalgia fugax have been identified. In this familiar syndrome hypertrophy of the IAS is present.

The treatment of proctalgia fugax is empirical. Spasmolytic suppositories, nitroglycerin sublingually, and inhalation of the beta-agonist salbutamol have been recommended.

Biliary System

9.1 Introduction

The bile produced in the liver is transported to the duodenum through the bile ducts. Bile mixes with the food bolus in the duodenum and facilitates digestion and absorption of certain nutrients. The liver produces bile at a constant volume, while bile is only required after a meal. Therefore, a storage system is present, which consists of the gallbladder. Whether bile is transported to the duodenum or the gallbladder is controlled in an elegant way, the volume of bile transported to the duodenum is dependent of the production in the liver, the contents and contraction of the gallbladder, and the contraction of the sphincter of Oddi. The bile ducts itself do not play a role in the regulation of bile transport as there is no peristalsis in these ducts.

9.2 Anatomy

Bile that is produced in the liver is released in the small bile ducts. These small bile ducts merge with other bile ducts and eventually end in the left or right hepatic duct and exit the liver (Fig. 9.1).

The right and left hepatic duct merges at the level of the liver hilum and together form the common hepatic duct. Further distally the cystic duct branches off and runs to the gallbladder. The hepatic duct is called common bile duct from that

point on. In the last few centimeters, the common bile duct runs through the pancreas and merges with the pancreatic duct. The point where the common bile duct and pancreatic duct merge and open in the duodenum is called papilla of Vater or major duodenal papilla (Fig. 9.2).

The sphincter of Oddi surrounds the most distal part of the common bile duct and pancreatic duct and controls the outflow of bile and pancreatic juices. The sphincter of Oddi consists of circular and longitudinal muscle layers, and the largest part of the sphincter is located within the duodenal wall.

9.3 Bile

The liver produces approximately 1 l bile every day. In fasting conditions the bile flows to the gallbladder, where it is stored until the next meal. When nutrients and fat in particular reach the duodenum, the hormone cholecystokinin (CCK) is released. This hormone stimulates hepatic bile production and promotes contractions of the gallbladder, which results in emptying of the gallbladder and flow of bile through the bile ducts into the duodenum. Bile is a mixture of bile salts, cholesterol, phospholipids, bile pigments, and water. Bile salts together with fat and fat-soluble contents from the foods form micelles that make the fat and fat-soluble contents soluble in water and allow absorption in the intestine. In case bile

© Springer International Publishing Switzerland 2016
A.J. Bredenoord et al., *A Guide to Gastrointestinal Motility Disorders*,
DOI 10.1007/978-3-319-26938-2_9

does not reach the bowel, for example, because of an obstruction of the bile ducts by a stone or tumor, much less fat absorption will take place. An absolute shortage of bile can occur after prolonged percutaneous drainage of the bile ducts.

The vast majority of bile produced in the bowel is absorbed again in the terminal ileum, and this is called the enterohepatic cycle. A patient can also develop a shortage of bile when a large part of ileum is missing, for example, after a large resection and reuptake of bile is not possible anymore.

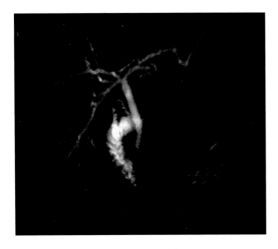

Fig. 9.1 Magnetic resonance cholangiopancreatography (MRCP) visualizes bile ducts and pancreatic duct

9.4   Gallbladder

The main function of the gallbladder is the storage of bile. Because the gallbladder also absorbs water from the bile, concentration of the bile takes place. Sometimes the gallbladder has been surgically removed, usually because of problems related to bile stones. This situation however does not result in problems in fat digestion and absorption.

The contractions of the gallbladder are related to its function. The muscles in the gallbladder wall contract, causing the bile to get squeezed out. The duration and force of the contractions are dependent on the concentration of fat in the ingested meal. High-fat meals require a lot of bile and result in the strongest gallbladder wall contractions.

In fasting conditions the migrating motor complex (MMC) controls motility of the small bowel but also the gallbladder. A 90-min cycle exists of motor quiescence (phase I), increasing motor activity (phase II) and a short period of strong contractions (phase III). In phase I the muscles of the gallbladder wall are relaxed and the pressure in the gallbladder is low. Most bile that is produced in the liver flows into the gallbladder, and only a small amount flows through the bile ducts into the duodenum. When the

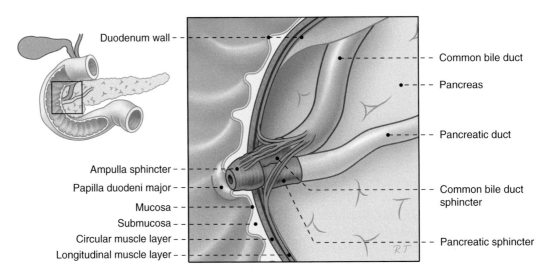

Fig. 9.2 Anatomy of the sphincter of Oddi (Published with kind permission of © Rogier Trompert Medical Art 2015)

bowels enter phase III, strong contractions of the gallbladder wall start causing bile to flow out of the gallbladder. At the end of phase III, the gallbladder relaxes again. Bile thus contributes chemical cleansing to the mechanical cleaning provided by the MMC.

9.5   Sphincter of Oddi

In addition to the contractility of the gallbladder, the sphincter of Oddi is also important in the regulation of bile flow into the duodenum. The sphincter will relax during and after a meal, so that the bile that is squeezed out of the gallbladder can flow easily into the duodenum. In the fasting state, the sphincter is contracted and exerts a tonical pressure that is higher than the pressure in common bile duct and duodenum. The pressure in the bile ducts will therefore increase and bile will preferentially flow toward the gallbladder.

In addition to the tonic pressure in the sphincter of Oddi, short phasic contractions are present in the sphincter that start proximally and move in distal direction. These phasic contractions push the contents of the sphincter toward the duodenum. These contractions also prevent the migration of intestinal bacteria into the bile ducts. The contractions of the sphincter of Oddi are influenced by several hormones and drugs (Table 9.1).

9.6   Regulation of Bile Flow into the Duodenum

As previously mentioned, the flow of bile into the duodenum is determined by the contractility of the gallbladder and the sphincter of Oddi. The contractility of gallbladder and sphincter of Oddi is controlled by hormones and neurons. During the initial phase of food intake, the gallbladder contractions are stimulated, and the sphincter activity are inhibited by a branch of the vagal nerve and through gastrin, released by the stomach. Once the food reaches the duodenum, cholecystokinin (CCK) is released by cells in the small

Table 9.1   Drugs that influence the sphincter of Oddi

Increase in sphincter pressure
Opiates (e.g., morphine)
Cholinergic agonists (e.g., nicotine)
Histamin-1-receptor agonists (e.g., betahistine)
Decrease in sphincter pressure
Nitrates
Glucagon
Calcium antagonists
Beta-adrenergic agonists (e.g., adrenalin)

bowel mucosa. Via the circulation CCK reaches and activates the gallbladder and sphincter of Oddi. CCK causes a strong contraction of the gallbladder and relaxation of sphincter, allowing the flow of bile into the duodenum. CCK also inhibits gastric emptying, causes a sensation of satiety, and stimulates the secretion of pancreatic juices.

9.7   Regulation of Flow of Pancreatic Juice into the Duodenum

The pancreas is a gland in the retroperitoneum. The pancreas has both an endocrine and exocrine function. The endocrine cells of the pancreas produce the hormones insulin, glucagon, and somatostatin and release these hormones in the circulation. The exocrine cells produce an alkaline fluid rich of bicarbonate and digestive enzymes. This alkaline fluid neutralizes the gastric acid that enters the duodenum. Most enzymes are secreted as inactive proenzymes and are later converted into active enzymes. The digestive enzymes play a role in the digestion of all types of foods. Trypsin and chymotrypsin facilitate digestion of proteins, lipases facilitate fat digestion, and amylase facilitates polysaccharides. The hormone secretin stimulates the secretion of the alkaline fluid, while CCK stimulates the secretion of the proenzymes. Both CCK and secretin are released from cells within the duodenum that are activated by luminal nutrients. The pancreatic duct merges with the common bile duct just before it ends in the duodenum. In the very last part of the pancreatic duct, it is surrounded by the sphincter of Oddi. This sphincter helps to regulate the flow of pancreatic juice into the duodenum and is probably also important in preventing duodenal content from entering the pancreatic duct.

9.8 Motility Disorders of the Bile Ducts and Gallbladder

9.8.1 Gallstones

The formation of bile stones is partly dependent on the constituents of bile and partly dependent on the motility of the gallbladder. In the gallbladder water is absorbed which results in concentration of the bile. Cholesterol is not soluble in water, but in bile it is dissolved in micelles of bile salts and phospholipids. If bile contains more cholesterol than can be dissolved in micelles, cholesterol crystals are formed. These crystals grow and become cholesterol stones, the most common type of gallstones. The bile is then oversaturated with cholesterol. Besides cholesterol stones, also bile salt or pigment stones exist. Conjugated bilirubin is water-soluble, but unconjugated bilirubin is not. Pigment stones arise from crystals of unconjugated bilirubin and are mainly formed in conditions with a high secretion of unconjugated bilirubin.

Besides cholesterol oversaturation, also infrequent or decreased emptying of the gallbladder plays a role. During pregnancy there is a decreased gallbladder contractility caused by progesterone. Also vagotomy leads to a decreased gallbladder emptying which promotes gallstone formation. Infrequent and decreased emptying of the gallbladder occurs during a period with strong weight loss and during parenteral feeding.

Approximately 10 % of the population has gallstones, with females twice as frequent as males. However, in the majority of subjects, the gallstones do not cause any symptoms. Only one out of the five subjects will develop symptoms. Asymptomatic gallstones are generally not treated. Typical symptoms caused by gallstones that obstruct gallbladder outflow are acute pain in the right upper abdomen, radiating to the back. Often, the pain is colicky in nature and is accompanied by nausea and vomiting, and the symptoms are triggered by meal consumption. After an attack the pain is completely gone. Although the symptoms of gallstones can be very characteristic, the presentation is not always so typical. Sometimes it can be difficult to judge whether the symptoms of a patient are indeed related to the gallstones or whether another problem is present.

Gallstones can also get into the common bile and cause obstruction. Typical symptoms are then pain, jaundice, and liver function abnormalities. When a gallstone gets stuck in the cystic duct, it will not cause jaundice, because the bile from the liver can still reach the duodenum.

9.8.2 Gallbladder Dysfunction

In a subset of patients with typical colicky biliary-type pain, no gallstones are found. When even very small stones or crystals, such as that can only be seen with endoscopic ultrasound, are absent, a diagnosis of gallbladder dysfunction is considered by some. This is a controversial entity, however. Believers would advocate that patients with gallbladder dysfunction can be identified by means of measurement of gallbladder emptying after a fat-containing meal or administration of CCK. The emptying of the gallbladder can be assessed by scintigraphy or by abdominal ultrasound. Demonstration of delayed postprandial gallbladder emptying would support the decision to perform cholecystectomy. However, most clinicians do not believe that gallbladder dysfunction is well-defined disorder and do not consider measurement of gallbladder emptying to be a relevant diagnostic tool.

9.8.3 Sphincter of Oddi Dysfunction

Since the sphincter of Oddi is an important regulator of the flow of bile and pancreatic juice, conditions that interfere with normal sphincter function might lead to biliary and pancreatic symptoms and signs.

Sphincter of Oddi dysfunction is a controversial entity, used for conditions with an outflow problem at the sphincter of Oddi. The disorder is controversial because its existence, hallmarked by a relationship between symptoms and increased pressure at the sphincter of Oddi, has never been convincingly proven and recent evidence shows treatment of increased pressure at the sphincter does not change symptoms. Indeed more and more physicians abandon diagnostics and treatment of sphincter of Oddi dysfunction.

The following conditions are distinguished:

- Sphincter of Oddi stricture: an anatomic abnormality of the sphincter of Oddi. Usually the stricture is the result of fibrosis after inflammation, pancreatitis, stone passage, or sphincterotomy. In case of a sphincter of Oddi stricture, there is a continuous increased pressure at the sphincter.
- Sphincter of Oddi dysfunction: a functional abnormality of the sphincter that leads to outflow obstruction. As will be discussed, sphincter of Oddi dysfunction is a controversial entity.

Sphincter of Oddi dysfunction is associated with two different clinical conditions: colicky biliary pain and recurrent acute pancreatitis. It is very difficult to identify sphincter of Oddi dysfunction as a cause of symptoms of a patient. Usually, the diagnosis is considered when there is biliary pain without any other demonstrable abnormality. This pain can occur after a cholecystectomy or persist after cholecystectomy. Supporting for the diagnosis are increased liver enzymes during pain and a dilated common bile

Table 9.2 Milwaukee classification of sphincter of Oddi dyskinesia

Type I	Patients with all three criteria:
	Pain with associated elevation of liver transaminases
	Dilated common bile duct (>10 mm on ultrasound or >12 mm on ERCP)
	Delayed outflow of contrast from the common bile duct
Type II	Patients with one or two of the above criteria
Type III	Patients with none of these criteria

duct. Microlithiasis should be excluded. Three types of sphincter of Oddi dyskinesia are distinguished (Table 9.2).

In the past sphincter of Oddi manometry was performed in order to diagnose sphincter of Oddi dysfunction. With this technique, pressures in both components of the sphincter (common bile duct sphincter and pancreatic sphincter) were measured during ERCP. However, the finding of an increased pressure and subsequent sphincterotomy did not result in symptom reduction in large trials. In addition, sphincter of Oddi manometry is associated with a substantial risk of acute pancreatitis. This risk is higher than that of ERCP carried out for other indications. For these reasons, sphincter of Oddi manometry has now been largely abandoned.

Nowadays many argue that sphincter of Oddi dysfunction does not exist. A relationship between symptoms and increased pressure at the sphincter of Oddi has never been convincingly proven, and recent evidence shows that treatment of increased pressure at the sphincter does not change symptoms. It is felt by many that types I and II merely represent undetected microlithiasis in the common bile duct and that type III is a functional disorder with unknown etiology. Therefore, more and more physicians abandon diagnostics and treatment of sphincter of Oddi dysfunction.

Index

© Springer International Publishing Switzerland 2016
A.J. Bredenoord et al., *A Guide to Gastrointestinal Motility Disorders*,
DOI 10.1007/978-3-319-26938-2